Welcome, lovely people, to *Stirring Slowly*. It is my absolute pleasure to write the foreword to this beautiful book and to introduce you to a gorgeous, vivacious Greek Cypriot girl – the wonderful Georgie Hayden. She is a bundle of joy and she cooks fantastically well, with diligence, restraint and good taste.

Most importantly, she writes super-solid recipes that you know are going to deliver every time.

I have the authority to say this because Georgie has worked with me for more than ten years now, and I can still remember the day this avalanche of energy first came bounding through the front door of our office, ready and raring to go. And I have to say, a decade later, just standing next to her makes you feel good about pretty much everything in life, which hopefully gives you an indication of just how much joy you're going to get from these recipes.

What Georgie has achieved in this book, and what is truly unique, is that she's got right to the heart of what makes cooking so profoundly important – its ability to help us destress and re-energise, to heal and calm, and as Georgie says on the cover, to restore and revive. She has tapped into this beautifully in both her introduction to the book, and also in the words that set the tone of each chapter and introduce you to her recipes.

Not many people focus on this side of cooking, and the incredible power food has to help us through a bad day or to help us celebrate a good day. Yet both of these things are so important. Going out and choosing your ingredients with love and care, putting them together with a positive frame of mind, and with a sense of excitement, knowing you're going to tuck into a gorgeous bowl of home-cooked grub, or even better, share it with the people you love – you can't beat that. It's about all the wonderful processes of cooking – peeling, tearing, drizzling, kneading, whisking, blending and, of course, stirring.

Georgie – I love you like a sister (and Jools wants to marry you!). I'm so proud of what you've achieved in this brilliant book. I'm impressed and charmed by its beauty and inspired by the incredible words and recipes that fill its pages. I can't wait to get a copy on my kitchen shelf.

To Peter and Archimedes.
My boys, my all.

'and this is the wonder that's keeping the stars apart
I carry your heart (I carry it in my heart)'
E. E. CUMMINGS

STIRRING SLOWLY

recipes to restore & revive

GEORGINA HAYDEN

SQUARE PEG, LONDON

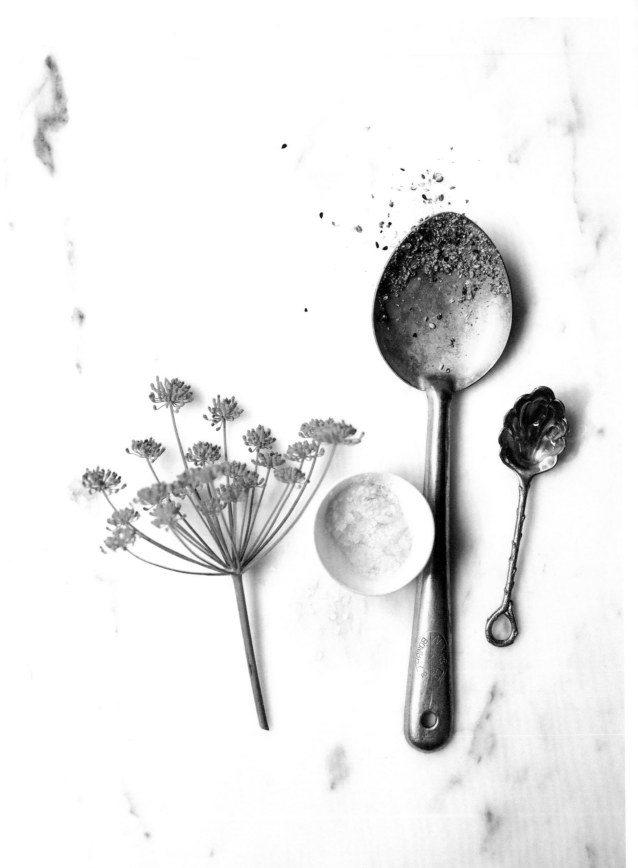

CONTENTS

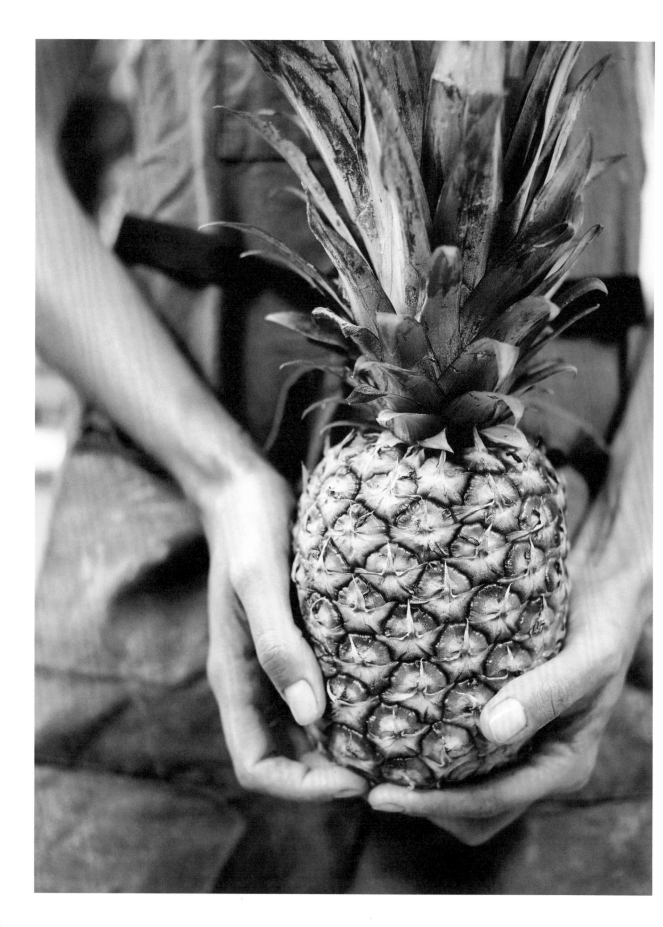

My earliest memories revolve around food.

That's not a total surprise given I spent the first year of my life – and then most weekends after that – living above my grandparents' restaurant in Tufnell Park. It was a classic family-run Greek Cypriot taverna, always noisy, always busy, and it was the heart of our family for many years. As kids, my sister and I would sit and pod peas, fill the salt and pepper shakers and occasionally cause chaos while my grandparents scurried around in the kitchen – it was always the most fun place to be. But my food memories go right back to when I was very little – and I'm surprised by how vivid they are. I can remember being taken in my buggy by my mum and sister to 'the smelly shop'. 'The smelly shop' was the most wonderful Italian deli, around the corner from the restaurant. It was filled with hanging salamis and cured meats, and every Saturday we'd make a pilgrimage. It had a multicoloured plastic strip curtain at the entrance, and when you walked in the smells were intoxicating – focaccia, olive oil, Parmesan, Parma ham – it was smelly, but in a good way. We loved it: it meant salami and honey sandwiches for lunch.

Growing up Greek Cypriot, family always came first. Three generations of my family would sit round the table together at least once a week. And in between we'd find any excuse for a get-together, be it big events like Greek Easter or just a proper barbecue. Whatever the occasion, there was – and still is – always food to match.

On Sundays it's a roast or, if the weather is good, souvla. Poorly? Avgolemono soup, olive-oil-soaked cotton wool in your ear and zivania (a potent Cypriot spirit) on your chest. Birthdays equal cakes; celebrations equal feasts; and if someone is unwell or unable to look after themselves, there is Tupperware filled with comforting meals for days.

With food at the centre of my childhood, perhaps it was inevitable I would end up working with it. As a teenager I started a farmers' market stall in north London selling platters of salads, homemade breads and painstakingly decorated cakes. Shortly after, I went to university to study Fine Art (I wanted to practise my obsession with styling on more than the cakes) and to this day I love sketching and photography. But when it came to choosing a career, food drew me back in. It wasn't a difficult decision – for me the kitchen has always felt like the most exciting place to be. And I still get to indulge my creative side, particularly now that the way food is visually presented gets more and more thought.

For the last ten years I've been incredibly lucky to work as part of Jamie Oliver's food team. There I develop, write and style recipes for books, magazine features, television and campaigns. Devising recipes is the highlight of my job and I get a real kick out of trying new things, understanding ingredients and figuring out dishes. But – no less important – along the way I have learnt about how and why people cook. Researching food traditions, learning about other food cultures, and simply observing what recipes strike a particular chord with readers all give me such a buzz.

So, while it goes without saying that how a dish tastes – and even how it looks – are important, I have realised over the years that these are only part of the picture. What truly brings food to life is the making, the eating, the sharing. Our restaurant days epitomised this; and, to this day, my yiayia's dishes have the same qualities. They may be rustic but that is, without a doubt, my favourite type of meal. They're made with love, they taste incredible and they feel like a symbol of family togetherness.

We all have an emotional attachment to food; it evokes memories, provides comfort and can often be a centre point in our day and lives.

It provides a break and a time to rest, socialize, restore and replenish. There are days when I am insanely busy and need a quick meal, but just because I don't have time doesn't mean I don't want to eat properly. And then there are days when I just want to stand in my kitchen and lose myself in baking, or preserving, or stirring something for hours on end. Food and flavour is important, but the process is key too. All I knew, when I started writing this book, was that I wanted to capture that – the entire process. The beauty, the deliciousness and the way cooking makes you feel.

Whether your life is going brilliantly right now or the opposite is true and you're having a hard time, we

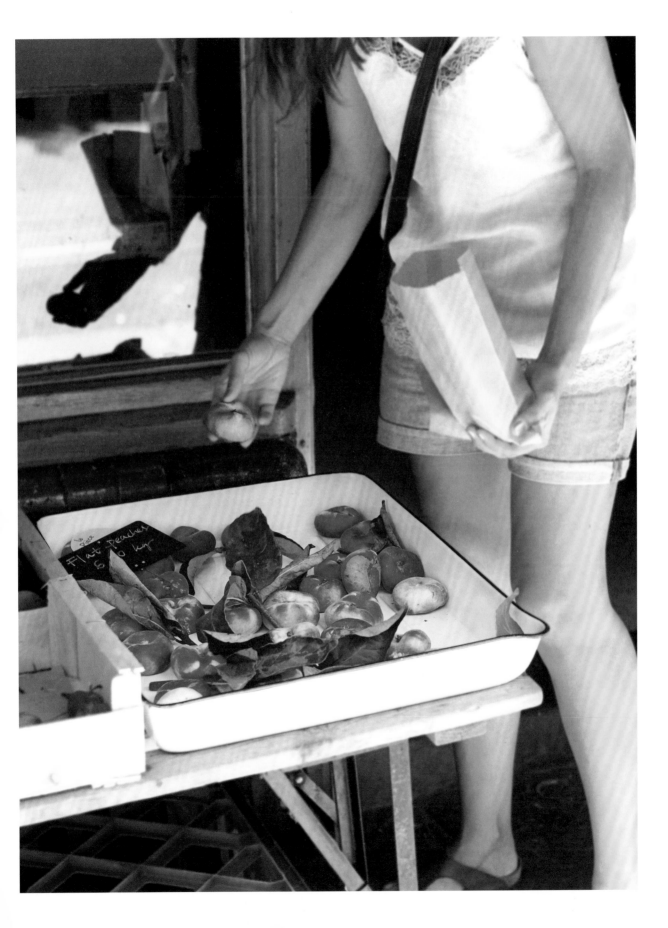

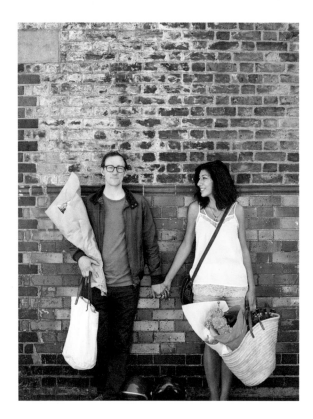

ruin scrambled eggs on toast when you cook for a living? Who knows, but I did.

After the scrambled egg incident, cooking went on to become an interesting and integral part of my healing journey. I wanted to focus on something I could control – I used cooking as a form of therapy. I decided to turn to the books from my groaning bookshelf and reteach myself to cook. Every Sunday I'd find recipes to make during the week, write a list, go to the shops and spend ages picking ingredients. It started out as a challenge, a way of getting into a routine, and in turn it helped rebuild my confidence and became fun.

The ingredients I used were nourishing, the process was relaxing and the eating was pure comfort.

all need to eat and food can play a huge part in any journey. I know that from experience. A couple of years ago my husband Pete and I had our lives turned upside down. After a heavenly pregnancy, our son Archie died just before birth and it felt like our world had fallen apart. Some days it feels like yesterday, other days it feels like so much has happened since then. That's the thing with grief and loss, it really isn't linear. But even in those early days when nothing felt OK, there were a few constants. And despite being the last things on our mind, we had to eat, we had to get through the day.

When Pete went back to work, he would come home at lunchtime every day to see me. It was then that I stepped into the kitchen for the first time since we'd lost Archie (we had survived on food from incredibly generous family and friends up until this point – something I will never forget). The plan was to make scrambled eggs and avocado on toast. Something so simple. In actual fact we pretty much just ate avocado. I burnt the toast and I ruined the eggs. How can you

Along the way there have been the meals that are nutritionally sound, such as mackerel and lentil salad (page 104), which I know are sorting me out on the inside. And there are recipes that take time and patience (the cakes, the breads, the pies) and there are the ones that are almost meditative (the gyozas on page 132 spring to mind – you could definitely practise some breathing techniques making those bad boys). Through cooking I have looked after myself, and my little family, and regained my strength and confidence.

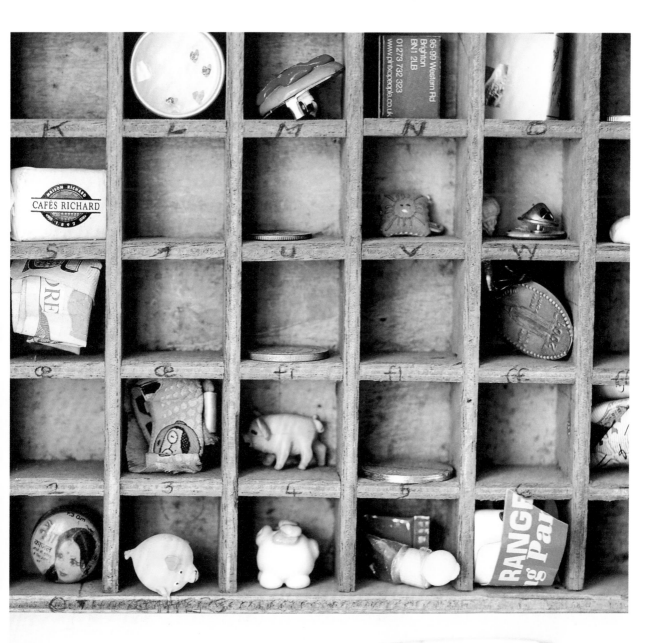

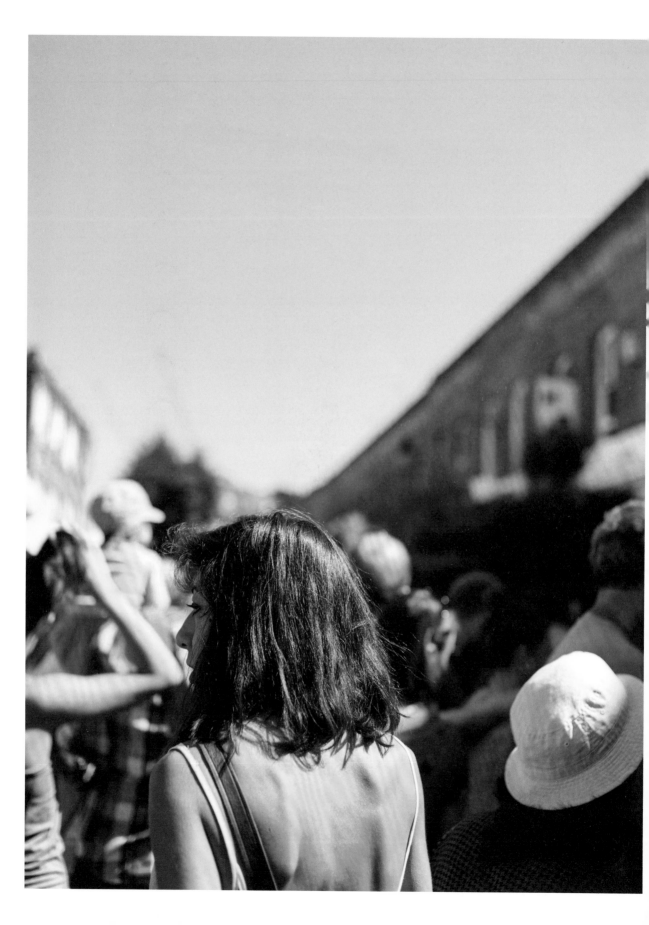

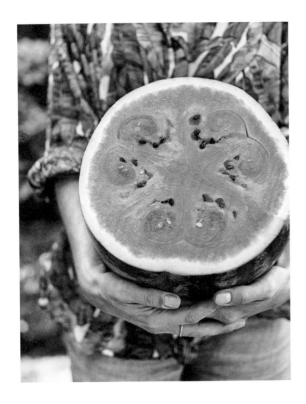

a decade, my diet is pretty well rounded. I'll now eat almost anything, but after years of a plant-based diet I do still turn to veg and fruit a lot of the time. I adore meat, and I love dairy (cheese beats cake for me, and pork wins every time), but I don't rely on them for every meal. I've been lucky enough to work with Jamie's nutritionist – Laura Matthews – for almost eight years now and she was kind enough to read the book for me. It's not calorie-counted but she's talked me through the health benefits of some of the recipes, either as a whole or by picking out key ingredients.

The current trend for healthy eating is great, and I'm sure it has made many of us a little more aware of what we put into our bodies.

But for me any meal that is made from scratch, lovingly, is good and clean.

Writing this book took time, and it has changed along the way – it isn't just a collection of my favourite meals, it has been a work in progress and I've lived it. The subtitle is 'recipes to restore and revive', as I believe this applies to us all. Maybe you've just had a bad day, or maybe you want a lifestyle that makes you feel amazing – whoever you are, the right food at the right time is hugely uplifting. I've thought hard what that means to me, and what it might mean to you.

In here you'll find breakfasts that make you want to get out of bed and won't weigh you down, soups that act as the edible equivalent of a warm hug, light week-night meals that are quick and nutritious, and heartier indulgent ones for when you want to relax. There is an all-important veg chapter, there are puddings and cakes that will leave you relaxed (and very popular), and, lastly, there are all the extra bits that make cooking, and eating, such a pleasure.

Having been vegetarian and pescatarian for almost

Cooking with raw ingredients is just as important as anything else. So much can be said through food. Sure, some foods are healthier, more nutritious, but surely the ones that aren't shouldn't be considered 'bad'; just more of a treat – it's all about balance. Often friends will ask what I'd like to eat if I'm invited round to dinner, and I will always say 'anything', because I genuinely feel that if someone is willing to take the time to make me something and cook for me, then that in itself is wonderful. I'll eat whatever they enjoy making. There is so much scope for pleasure in making, sharing and eating food. Whatever my day looks like – food is always a highlight.

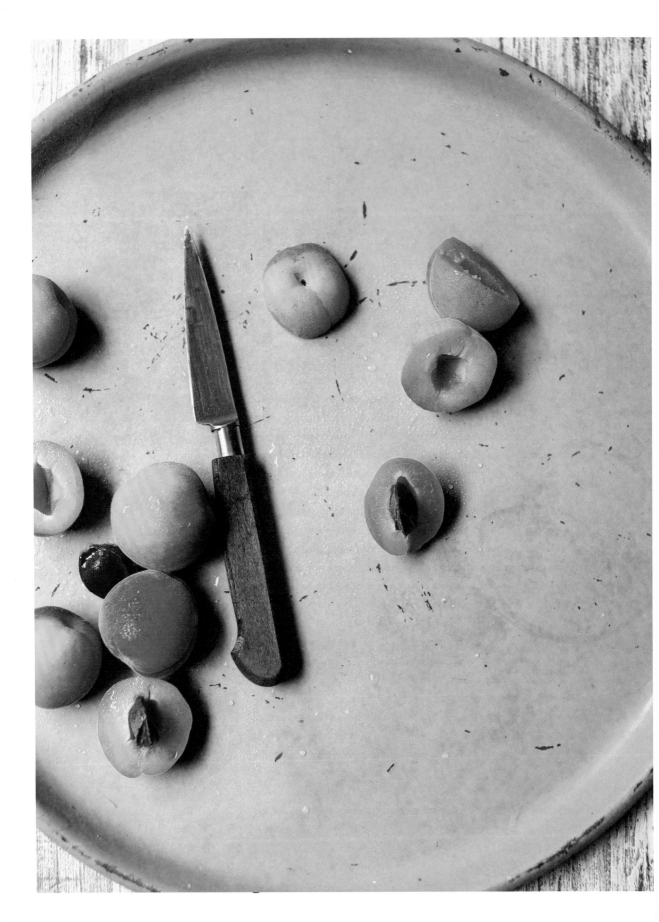

For recipes that are hopefully everyday, the ingredients should be easy to get hold of, while still being interesting and inspiring.

I spent a lot of time browsing the aisles of supermarkets when writing this book, as it felt important that the recipes I wrote were accessible and achievable. As I like to cook quite spontaneously according to how I feel, I tried to reflect that with ingredients everyone can pick up easily despite busy lives. There may be a handful of recipes where you'll need to search a little harder for things, depending on where you live. But I have tried to make sure that this has been kept to a minimum, and that worst case scenario, everything is available online.

FRUIT AND VEG
—

Fruit and veg It's obvious, but of course fruit and veg tastes better when it's in season; why have bland strawberries in winter that have travelled thousands of miles, when you can have flavourful, locally grown ones in the summer? I try to cook seasonally as much as I can – it means I get the best out of my meals and look forward to what's in season. Visit your local market or greengrocer to see what's in and plan your meals around that; you'll be rewarded with tasty produce that is less expensive too.

Lemons I always buy unwaxed lemons, as I love using their zest. If you buy waxed ones, simply pop them into a colander and pour over very hot or boiling water to remove the wax. You can do this for any waxed citrus fruit.

Salad Try to stay away from the pre-packed mixed salad bags – they are over-priced and lack flavour. Invest in a salad spinner, and buy heads of lettuce where possible.

Herbs You'll find that bunches tend to be larger and cheaper at your greengrocer's, so shop locally when you can. Also, my mum swears that soft herbs bought from greengrocer's and continental shops taste better and have more flavour than from the supermarkets and, dare I say it, I think she may be right.

Chillies One of my favourite tips my boss taught me is to store chillies in the freezer so I like to buy in bulk. They're an ingredient I use in abundance. Frozen, they become incredibly versatile; you can finely grate them over salads, eggs, veg – almost anything – to add a wonderful well-distributed heat.

MEAT AND FISH
—

Meat I firmly believe that the better the quality of meat you buy, the better your dish will taste. Of course buy the best you can afford, but with so many butchers and supermarkets stocking higher-welfare produce now you'd be hard pushed not to find good meat at a decent price. I like to know where my meat has come from and that it has had a good life, and if this means eating less of it but better quality, then that's fine by me. Also, if possible, try to buy locally, as opposed to imported.

Cheaper cuts of meat Keep an eye out for special offers on things like beef shin, lamb shoulder, lamb shanks, pork shoulder, chicken thighs... anything that requires slow cooking; they will freeze perfectly well for a few months, without losing flavour.

Fish Try to buy fish with an MSC (Marine Stewardship Council) logo, as you can be assured it has been responsibly sourced. If in doubt ask your fishmonger, as s/he'll be up to date with which fish are endangered and which are in abundance. The list is ever changing! So it is always good to ask.

EGGS
—

All eggs listed in this book are large – this is especially important if you are following any of the baking recipes. And ideally they should be free-range organic.
I store my eggs at room temperature – they're better for baking with and are less likely to crack when boiling.

DRY INGREDIENTS
—

When you first start cooking it can seem overwhelming how much you need to buy, but once you have a well-stocked store cupboard up and running, it becomes a lot more manageable and you won't have to run to the shops for everything. My store cupboard consists of a range of oils (extra virgin olive oil, groundnut oil and rapeseed oil are my heroes) and vinegars (white wine, red wine and cider). Tinned items such as tomatoes (always plum), coconut milk and lentils are a must. Dry produce such as a range of pastas, rice, lentils and beans. And much to the despair of my husband I also have a lot of condiments. I love chutneys, pickles, jams and mustards. There is a place for all of them in my cooking.

Then there are the dried herbs and spices. One tip I

highly recommend is to buy these from continental and ethnic shops, as they will be a fraction of the price compared to those you buy in little glass jars in supermarkets. They come in large bags and are easily stored in your own storage jars, or just resealed at the top once opened.

I have a whole range of flours and sugars, but if you aren't a keen baker these are less important – plain flour is all you need. I just like to be prepared, as you never know when you'll need to whip up a batch of blondies at the last minute.

Salt This hero ingredient deserves its own paragraph, just as a note with regard to my recipes. I use flaked sea salt in all my cooking, and where a specific amount is given this is to be taken into account. If you are using a fine sea salt you will need less – the salt grains are much smaller and you will therefore get more for your measure. Halve the amount given and season to taste from there.

OVEN
—

All recipes have been tested in a conventional electric oven. If you are using a fan or convection oven, adjust the temperature according to the instruction guide. Better yet, place an oven thermometer inside – this will give you the most accurate reading possible.

EQUIPMENT
—

I take pride in my 'kit', having spent years accumulating pots, pans and the like; however, it is surprisingly gadget-less. You don't need a million gadgets to be a good cook; spend your money on quality equipment and you'll instantly be in a better place. A sharp set of knives is a must. Using a sharp knife after having a blunt one feels like putting on a pair of glasses with the right prescription – it suddenly all makes sense. Wooden or plastic chopping boards only – the glass ones make me weep a little. A large, solid mortar and pestle is a thing of beauty (ours is rarely empty), as is a good peeler – I still can't peel potatoes quite like my yiayia, with just a little kitchen knife. A selection of saucepans and frying pans, in a range of sizes. Sometimes I am cooking for one, often for many – my collection reflects that. A good cast-iron casserole dish is fantastic – these can be used on the hob or in the oven and look gorgeous at the table. And one of my favourites – a good grater. Box graters are fine for coarse grating, but the hand-held fine graters that are available are just brilliant, they make grating citrus and hard cheese an absolute joy. Then there are measuring spoons, tongs, whisks, wooden spoons – the list goes on. Just be weary of faddy items; chances are they'll end up shoved to the back of your cupboard gathering dust in no time.

In terms of electrical kit, I don't have much. I have just four things. Two blenders (upright and hand-held), a food processor and a free-standing mixer. The selection of 'must-have' gadgets out there is overwhelming, but I guarantee you there isn't much else you really need. A good upright blender for smoothies, sauces and purées. A stick/hand-held blender for hot soups – hot soup in an upright blender is an accident waiting to happen. A food processor for chopping and blitzing is a must – breadcrumbs, veg, even cake mixes. Also, depending on the type you go for, they often come with slicing and grating attachments, which I love. Never has making a gratin or slaw been so easy. And lastly a free-standing mixer. They aren't cheap, but an electric hand whisk is a great and inexpensive alternative. If you really are a keen baker, though, it's definitely an item worth investing in.

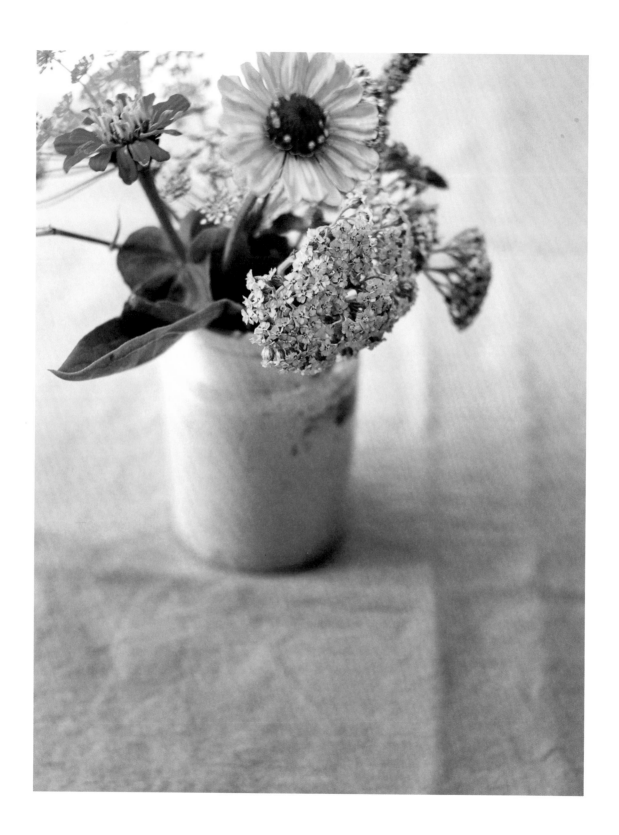

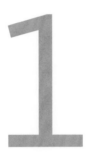

A SUNNY START TO THE DAY

—

I used to be more of a breakfast avoider than a breakfast lover, but now it has become the reason I get out of bed most mornings. No matter how busy life gets, there is always time to sit at the table with a pot of coffee, juice and a proper breakfast; I love our morning ritual. Here I have included recipes for quick and nutritious weekday breakfasts, prepare-ahead ideas, and long leisurely brunches. Because breakfast really is the most important, and exciting, meal of the day.

SLOW-COOKED PINHEAD PORRIDGE

This is porridge but on another level. It is insanely creamy, to the point where you'll think there has to be butter or cream in it, but there is nothing naughty in this addictive breakfast bowl. What you do need is time – you can't rush it, this is literally meant to be stirred slowly. However, a great tip is to make a large batch of this on a Sunday, when most of us have more time (I do not have 45 minutes to spare on a weekday morning, you're lucky if I brush my hair), as it keeps really well. Just cool it down, store it in the fridge and reheat it with a splash of milk and water – works a treat. You can obviously serve it how you like – straight up with a little brown sugar is heavenly – but here is the way I like to eat mine.

SERVES 4

—

75g rolled oats

50g pinhead oatmeal

700ml milk *(please use full-fat or semi-skimmed, skimmed is too watery)*

½ teaspoon sea salt

2 bananas

½ teaspoon ground cinnamon

1 tablespoon poppy seeds

3–4 tablespoons honey or light soft brown sugar

Place the oats and oatmeal in a large saucepan with the milk, salt and 300ml of water. Pop on to a medium heat and slowly bring to the boil. As soon as it starts to boil, turn the heat down to a simmer and leave the porridge to gently bubble away for around 35-40 minutes, stirring often so it doesn't stick, and becomes thick and creamy. If it feels like it is thickening up too much, add a splash more water or milk.

Peel and slice the bananas. Finish the porridge by stirring in the cinnamon and poppy seeds, and ladle into bowls. If I'm using honey I like to drizzle it into the bowl before ladling in the porridge; if I'm using sugar I sprinkle it over the porridge and leave it to melt into a pool of caramel, swirl it in, then scatter over the sliced bananas.

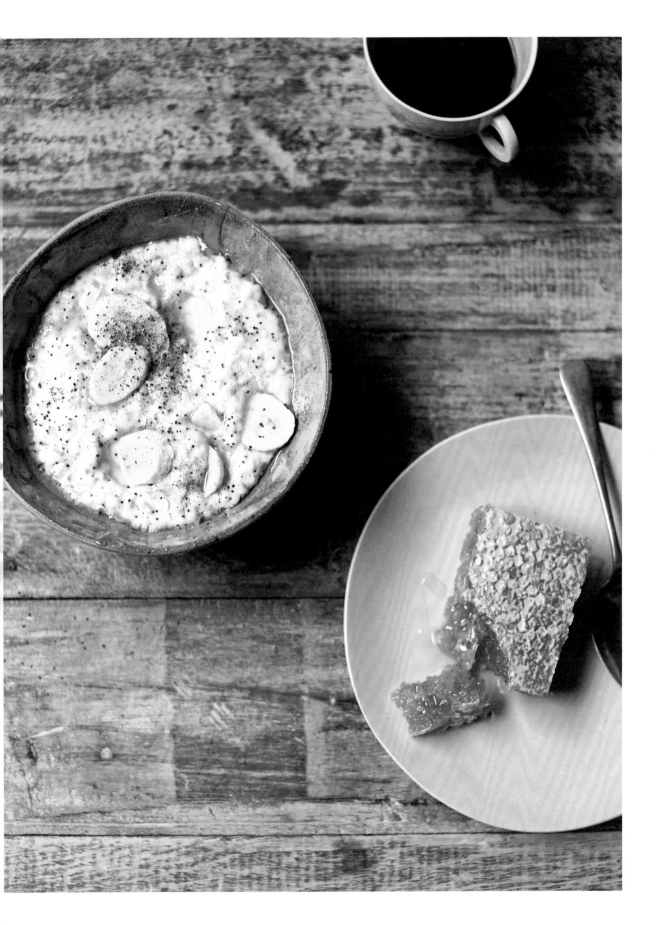

QUICK FLAPJACK CHERRY GRANOLA

As with many great things in life, this recipe was created by accident, and stemmed from curiosity and a little bit of laziness. My husband, Pete, has a nut allergy, which means that most shop-bought granolas and mueslis are out of the question, so I'll often make him a batch with just seeds and dried fruit. However, after much promising but not much making, one morning we found ourselves with an abundance of fresh fruit and some delicious yoghurt but no granola (fruit and yoghurt alone is just not enough in this house) – so I got playing and this pan-fried quick granola was created. And you know what? It's delicious: chewy like a flapjack and a little crunchy like a granola, it's easy to make and a great alternative to the oven-made stuff.

SERVES 4
—

1 tablespoon olive oil *(or any flavourless oil)*

1 teaspoon vanilla extract

125g rolled porridge oats

50g dried cherries or cranberries

50g dried figs *(or any other dried fruit you like – dates and apricots work well)*

2 tablespoons mixed seeds *(pumpkin, sesame, poppy, sunflower)*

a pinch of sea salt

¼ teaspoon ground cinnamon

3 tablespoons runny honey

a punnet of your favourite mixed berries, to serve

homemade yoghurt, to serve *(see page 238)*

Drizzle the oil and vanilla extract into a medium-size non-stick pan with a splash of water and place it on a medium heat. Scatter in the oats and stir it all together. Pop on the lid and leave the oats to cook for 5 minutes. Meanwhile, roughly chop the cherries and chop the figs (or whichever fruit you are using) into similar-size pieces.

When the oats have had a chance to soften, remove the lid and add the seeds to the pan. Turn the heat up a little and toast the oats and seeds for a couple of minutes. Sprinkle in the salt and add the chopped dried fruit and cinnamon. Toss everything together and drizzle over the honey. Cook for 2-3 minutes until you have a golden chewy granola that's a little crisp around the edges.

Leave in the pan for a few minutes to cool, then spoon over fresh fruit and yoghurt or leave to cool completely, and store in a sealed jar until needed.

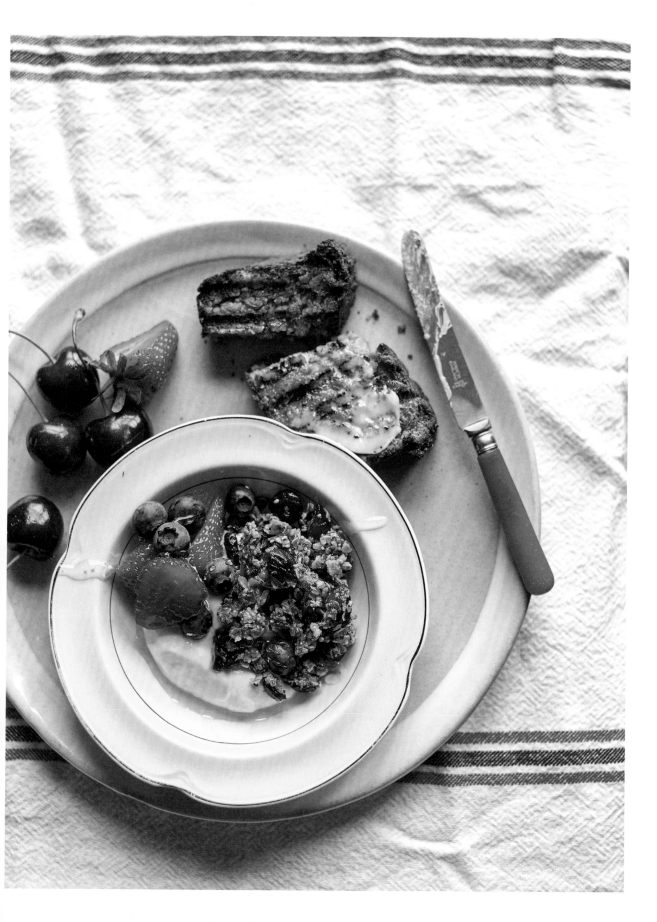

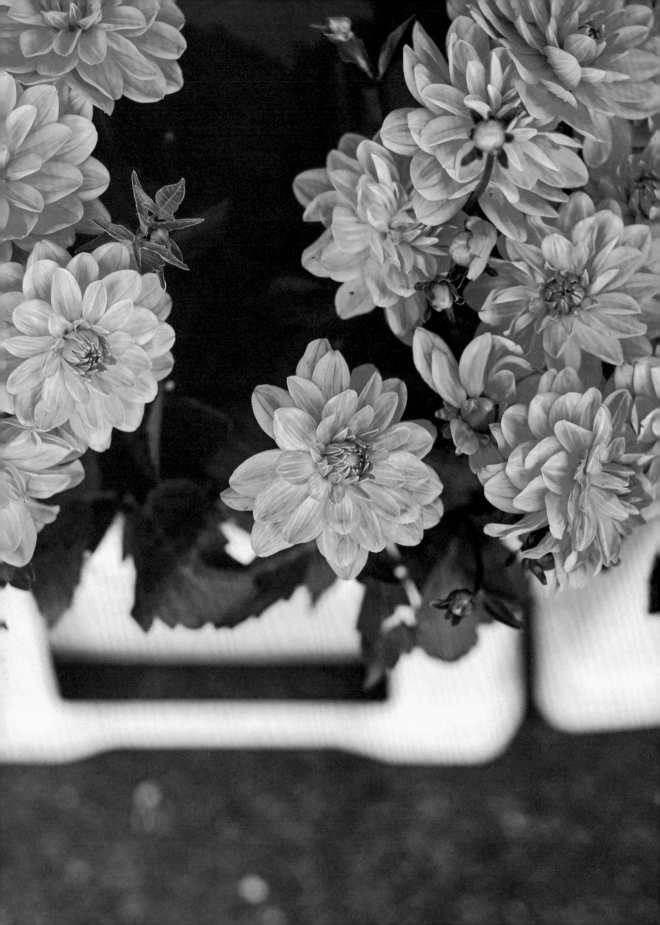

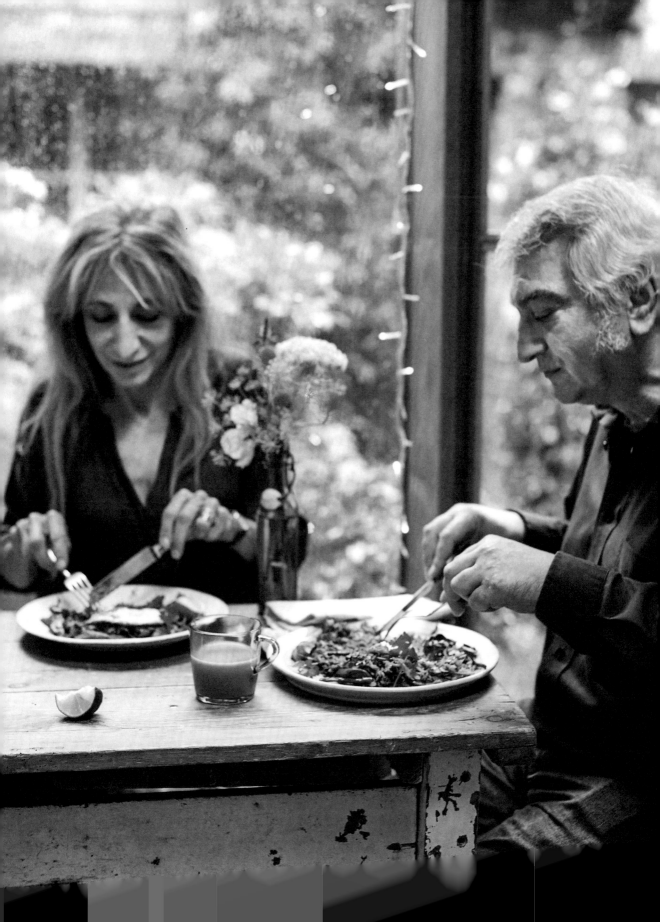

GRIDDLED FRUIT SALAD WITH HONEY GINGER DRESSING

I love serving fruit this way. It's great on its own, with yoghurt, granola or even as a pud (it looks wonderful when served on a platter with a bowl of whipped cream and meringues). Also, you can treat the recipe as a guide and use whatever fruits you have to hand – you can griddle any firmer fruits successfully.

SERVES 2 (multiply as needed)

—

1½ teaspoons sesame seeds

a 1cm piece of ginger

2 tablespoons honey

1 lime

1 nectarine or peach

1 apricot

1 pear

¼ of a pineapple

a handful of blueberries

Place a griddle pan on a high heat, and leave to get hot while you prepare the dressing. Scatter the sesame seeds into a small saucepan or frying pan and toast until lightly golden over a low heat, then remove from the pan and leave to one side.

Peel the ginger. Squeeze the honey into the frying pan, finely grate in the ginger and the lime zest, and squeeze in the lime juice. Place on a medium-low heat, and gently stir it all together. Bring to a gentle boil, then reduce the heat and simmer for 2 minutes. Remove from the hob and leave to one side.

Prepare your fruit for griddling. Halve the nectarine or peach, remove the stone and cut each piece in half again. Halve the apricot and remove the stone. Trim the pear and cut in half, then in half again, so you have 4 wedges. Peel the pineapple, cut away the core and chop into rough pieces, around 2–3cm in size.

Place all the cut fruit on the hot griddle (you will probably have to do this in two batches), and turn them so they get charred on all sides. Transfer to a bowl or platter and scatter over the blueberries. Drizzle over the honey ginger dressing, gently toss through, and finish by scattering over the toasted sesame seeds. Serve straight away.

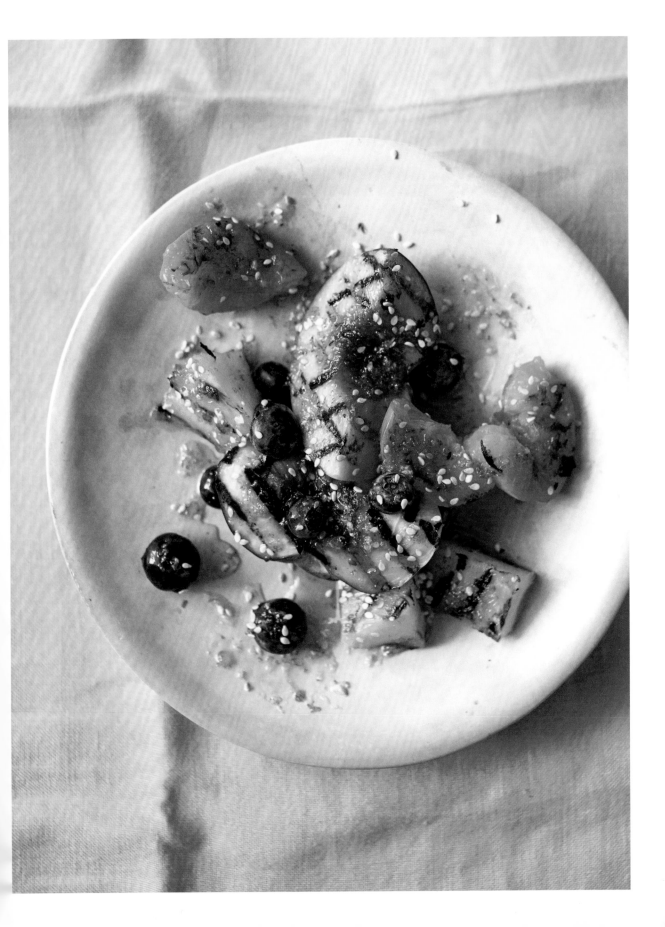

CARAMELISED APPLE, RICOTTA AND HAZELNUT PANCAKES

Pancakes are a big weekend hit in our house, with toppings and mixes constantly being tweaked depending on what's in season. Berries in the summer, citrus in the winter, savoury any time. But one of my favourites is this tarte Tatin-style pancake, because it (kind of) makes it acceptable to eat one of my favourite puddings for breakfast. And it isn't as naughty as it tastes.

SERVES 4
—

50g toasted hazelnuts

2 nice eating apples *(I like Cox's or Braeburn, nothing with a waxy skin)*

1 orange

250g ricotta

2 large eggs

1 teaspoon vanilla extract

175ml milk

125g wholemeal flour

1 teaspoon baking powder

a pinch of salt

groundnut oil

4 tablespoons maple syrup

Greek yoghurt, to serve

Place the nuts in a food processor and blitz to a slightly coarse consistency. Slice each apple into 6 thin slices, then place in a bowl and finely grate over the orange zest. Spoon the ricotta into a sieve and press out any excess liquid, then transfer it to a large mixing bowl. Separate the eggs, placing the whites into a clean mixing bowl and the yolks in with the ricotta. Beat the vanilla and milk in with the ricotta. Then add the flour, baking powder, salt and most of the chopped hazelnuts. Mix until just combined.

Whisk the egg whites with an electric whisk (or elbow grease) until you have stiff peaks. Fold one spoonful into the ricotta to loosen, then fold through the rest of the egg whites, keeping the mixture as light as possible.

Using a pastry brush or some kitchen paper, rub a large non-stick frying pan with an thin, even layer of groundnut oil. Pop on to a medium heat and lay out 6 of the apple slices. Halve the orange and squeeze over the juice from one half. Lightly cook the apples for 2-3 minutes then flip them all over. Top each slice with a large spoonful of the ricotta batter, using half of the batter between 6 slices. Reduce the heat a little and gently cook the pancakes for 6-8 minutes, giving the batter enough time to set. Carefully flip the pancakes over and cook for a further 4-5 minutes, until cooked through.

Finish by drizzling with 2 tablespoons of maple syrup, flipping them back over for a minute so the apples become caramelised. Serve straight away, with a dollop of yoghurt, a sprinkle of the reserved chopped hazelnuts and extra maple syrup on the side. Wipe the pan clean then repeat with the remaining apple slices and batter.

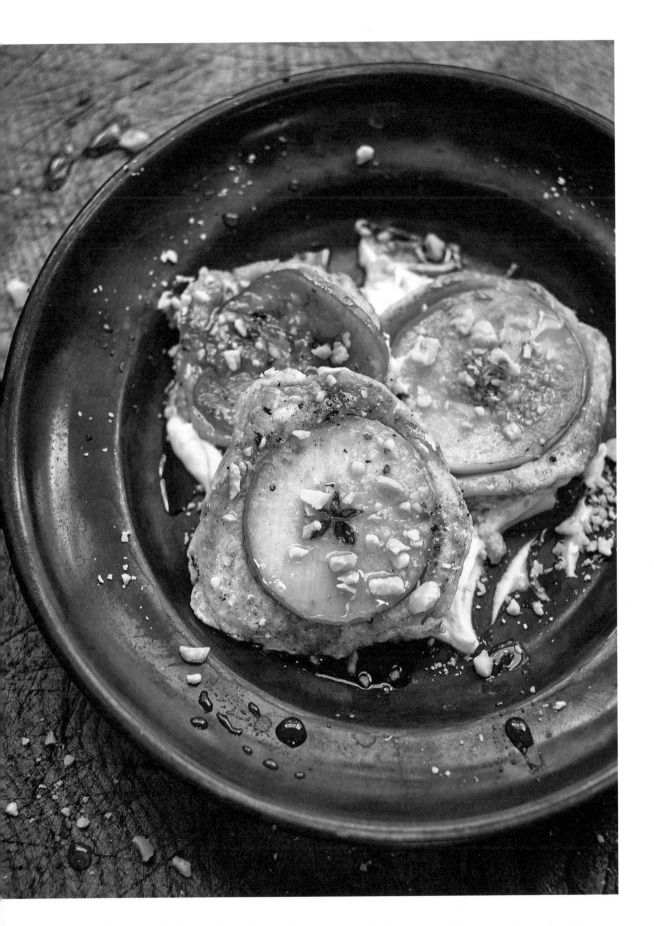

WHOLEGRAIN NASI GORENG WITH SPINACH

On honeymoon in Indonesia this was our breakfast of choice. Nasi goreng is a cracking start to the day, it's a good source of protein, and the ingredients I have used here mean it releases energy slowly. (Think kedgeree and you're on the right page.) Tastes even better after a slightly late night, too... Heck, it's great at any time.

SERVES 2 (Multiply/halve as needed)

—

125g brown basmati rice

a few sprigs of coriander

2 garlic cloves

2 shallots

1 red chilli

a 2cm piece of ginger

100g green beans

100g baby leaf spinach

groundnut oil

¼ teaspoon turmeric

2 tablespoons kecap manis *(if you can't find kecap manis, replace with soy sauce and a tablespoon of runny honey)*

1 tablespoon low-salt soy sauce

2 large eggs

sea salt and freshly ground black pepper

1 lime, halved

sriracha, or other chilli sauce, to serve

Cook the rice according to the packet instructions and leave to cool. To cool it quickly, spread it out on a tray. (If you can cook your rice and chill it the night before, it'll be even better.)

Prep all your veg and then you'll be ready to go. Pick the coriander leaves and roughly chop; leave them to one side for later. Peel the garlic and shallots, and finely slice along with the chilli (deseeded if you don't want it too hot) and the coriander stalks. Peel the ginger and slice into fine matchsticks. Trim the green beans, roughly chop into 2–3cm pieces, and roughly chop the spinach.

Place a medium-size saucepan of salted water on to boil and blanch the green beans in the boiling water for 3 minutes. Remove with a slotted spoon and plunge into cold water. If you are serving with poached eggs, turn the heat down under the pan, so the water is ready to poach the eggs in later on. If you are serving with fried eggs, take the pan off the heat and place a medium frying pan on the hob.

Pop another large non-stick frying pan or wok on a medium heat and pour in a drizzle of oil. Add the finely sliced shallots and sauté for 5 minutes, then add the sliced garlic, chilli, ginger, and coriander stalks. Soften for a further 5 minutes, then add the turmeric and drained beans. Fry for 2 minutes, then add the chilled rice, kecap manis and soy sauce. Fry everything for 5 minutes, until the rice is piping hot, stirring frequently. At the same time, cook your eggs to your liking – I fry/poach mine for just under 3 minutes, for a runny yolk. Finish the rice by stirring through the chopped spinach and coriander, and then season to taste.

Plate up the nasi goreng, top with an egg and any leftover coriander. Serve with a lime half on the side, and a bottle of sriracha for the table.

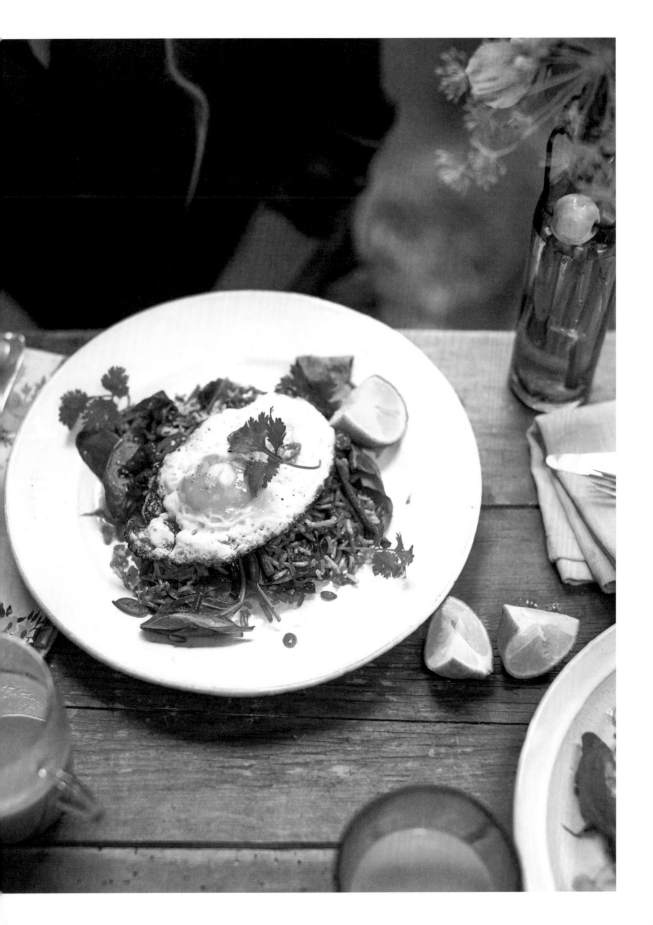

BOMBAY OMELETTE

I had my first masala omelette on a trip to India and it totally converted me to eating punchy flavours in the morning. Breakfast in India isn't a sweet affair – no sugary cereals or cakes, but spicy masala omelettes, dosas with sambal, meals that really will set you up for the day and don't weigh you down. This is now a go-to dish in our house, and not just at breakfast time – it will often get made in the evening if we're hungry and tired. It's incredibly straightforward and easily adaptable, depending on what you have to hand. A perfect protein-packed start to the day.

SERVES 2 (multiply/halve as needed)
—

½ a red onion

2 small vine tomatoes

½ a bunch of coriander

1 green chilli

4 large eggs

30g baby spinach leaves

½ teaspoon ground turmeric

½ teaspoon garam masala

½ teaspoon ground cumin

sea salt and freshly ground black pepper

½ a lemon

2 knobs of butter

Peel and finely chop the onion. Halve the tomatoes, scoop out the seeds with a teaspoon and discard, then finely chop the flesh. Finely chop the coriander stalks and leaves. Halve the chilli, deseed and finely slice. Whisk the eggs together until well combined, then season generously and whisk in the onion, tomatoes, coriander, chilli, turmeric, garam masala and cumin. Put the spinach leaves into a bowl, squeeze just enough lemon to coat, toss together, then leave to one side.

Melt half the butter in a medium non-stick frying pan over a medium heat and ladle in half the omelette mixture. Swirl the eggs around for 2 minutes, pushing them to the middle and tilting the pan so that all the mixture has a chance to set. Leave it for a minute, then slip the omelette on to your serving plate. Top with half the dressed spinach and fold the omelette in half. Serve straight away, and repeat with the remaining butter, omelette mix and spinach.

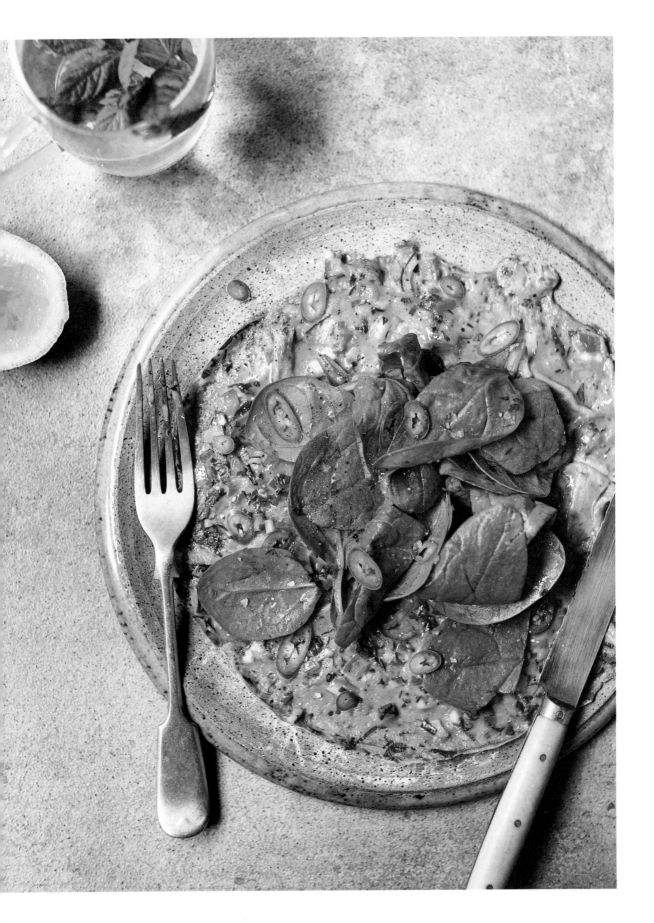

MENEMEN WITH LEMON-ROASTED FETA AND OLIVES

Menemen is a fabulous Turkish breakfast of velvety scrambled eggs in softened tomatoes and peppers. We grew up eating the Cypriot version (without the peppers) at all times of the day. Instead of scrambling the eggs into the veg I often coddle them, as I've done here. But if you want to try the original version, simply whisk the eggs and very gently scramble them through at the end.

SERVES 4

—

150g feta

1 lemon

12 black olives

½ a bunch of oregano

olive oil

sea salt and freshly ground black pepper

2 Middle Eastern peppers, red and green *(or just regular ones will be fine)*

2 onions

1 green chilli

5 ripe tomatoes

1 tablespoon tomato purée

4 large eggs

a few sprigs of flat-leaf parsley, leaves picked

a good pinch of Turkish chilli flakes (optional) *(regular dried chilli flakes are fine too)*

flatbread or pitta, to serve

Preheat the oven to 200°C/gas 6. Place the feta into a small dish and finely grate over the lemon zest. Destone and roughly chop the olives. Pick the oregano leaves and toss half of them with the olives, then scatter over the feta. Cut the lemon into 4 wedges and tuck into the dish. Drizzle everything with a little olive oil, season, and pop into the oven for 20 minutes, or until everything is golden and crisp around the edges.

Meanwhile halve and deseed the peppers, and chop into 1cm pieces. Peel and finely slice the onions and deseed and finely slice the chilli. Place a large non-stick frying pan on a medium-low heat with 3 tablespoons of olive oil. Add the veg and the rest of the oregano and sauté for 10 minutes, until softened but not coloured. While the veg are cooking, peel the tomatoes. Score a little cross on the top of each one, then place them in a large jug or bowl and cover with just-boiled water. Leave them for a minute, then drain from the water, carefully peel away the skin and finely chop the flesh. When the veg are have softened, stir in the tomato purée, fry for a minute, then add the chopped tomatoes and all their juices. Season well and cook for a further 10 minutes, adding a splash of water if needed, until the veg have cooked down and thickened.

When the veg have thickened, use a spoon to create 4 pockets in the mixture. Crack an egg into each pocket and cook for 5 minutes, then cover with the lid and cook for 5 minutes more, until the whites are cooked through but the yolks are nice and runny (unless you don't like runny yolks, in which case cook for a few more minutes).

Roughly chop the parsley leaves, and when the menemen is ready, sprinkle it over the top and crumble over the roasted feta and olives. Sprinkle them over the dried chilli if using, and serve with toasted flatbreads or pitta and the charred lemon wedges.

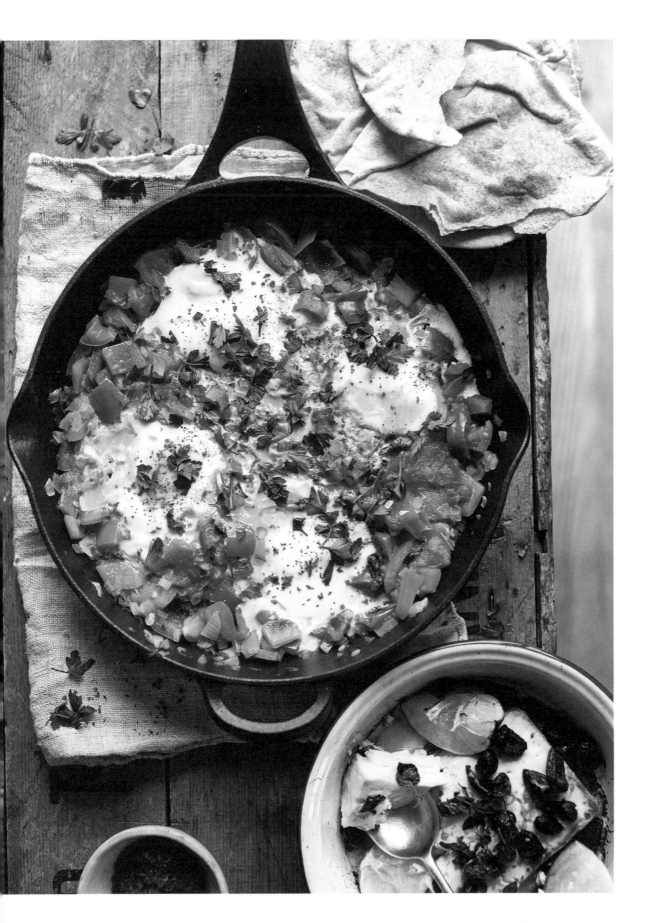

KIPPER HASH WITH WATERCRESS YOGHURT AND GRIDDLED CUCUMBER

We know we should be eating more oily fish, and kipper ticks a lot of the boxes. It's packed with omega-3 - great for the heart and helping reduce heart disease, and it's a good source of vitamin D which we need to absorb calcium. Start with an incredible breakfast and chances are you'll continue to eat well for the rest of the day.

SERVES 4

—

4 kipper fillets *(around 280g in total)*

500ml milk

600g floury potatoes, such as Maris Pipers

½ a bunch of chives

4 spring onions

sea salt and freshly ground black pepper

a 1cm piece of fresh horseradish or 1 teaspoon jarred grated horseradish

1 lemon

olive oil

½ a cucumber

100g watercress

200g Greek yoghurt

Place the kipper fillets in a large frying pan and pour over the milk. Place on a medium heat and gently bring to the boil. As soon as the milk starts to boil, reduce the heat to low, simmer for 6 minutes, then remove from the hob and leave to one side to cool. When the kippers are cool enough to handle, discard most of the milk and gently flake the fish, discarding the skin and as many bones as you can.

While the kippers are poaching, chop the potatoes into even-size pieces and place in a pan of cold salted water. Bring to the boil over a medium heat and when it starts to bubble, reduce the heat slightly and boil the potatoes for around 12 minutes, or until cooked through. (You can peel the potatoes if you like, but I love the texture of crispy potato skins.) Drain and leave to steam dry in the colander for a few minutes so there is no water left on them. Return the potatoes to the dry pan and mash with a potato masher until mostly smooth.

Finely chop the chives, and add to the mashed potatoes with the flaked kippers and a splash of the poaching milk. Trim and finely slice the spring onions and add to the pan along with a good pinch of salt and pepper. Peel and finely grate in the horseradish and finely grate in the lemon zest. Mix everything together well, with your hands if you want, making sure it's well combined.

Place a griddle pan on a high heat. Clean the pan you poached the kippers in and pop it on to a medium heat; pour in a good glug of olive oil. Spoon in the potato mixture and flatten it out with a spatula so it is around 2cm thick. Fry for around 12–15 minutes, turning over parts of the hash here and there, to get a lovely golden crust forming throughout. It's ready when the underside is crispy, while also having a good crust on top. »

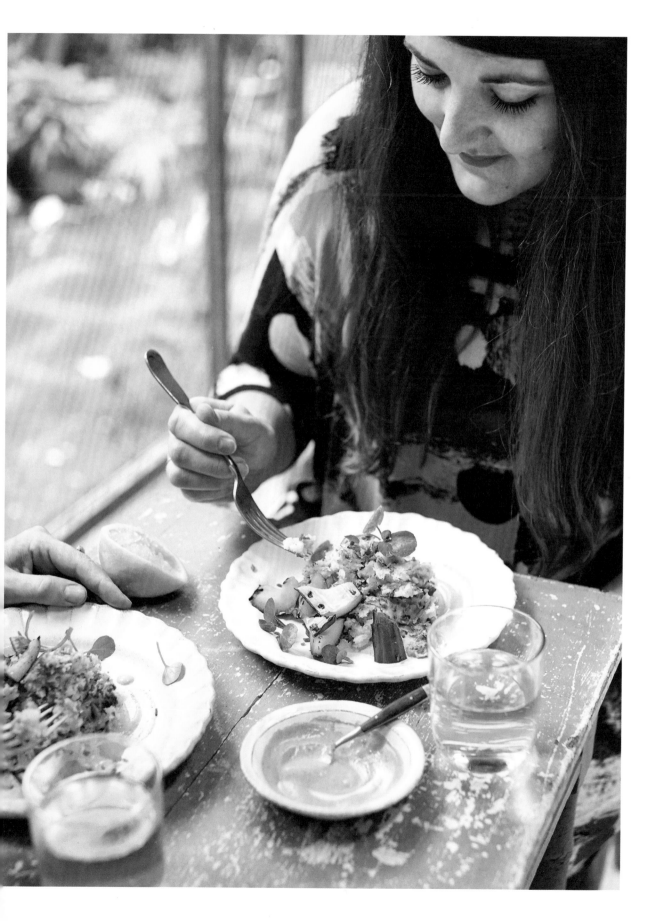

« While the hash is frying, cut the cucumber in half lengthways, and each piece in half again so you end up with 4 long wedges. Scoop out the seeds with a teaspoon and pop the cucumber pieces on to the hot griddle. Grill for a few minutes on each side, so that you have good char marks all over.

Pop 70g of the watercress into a blender with the juice of ½ the lemon, a pinch of salt and pepper and the Greek yoghurt. Blitz until smooth.

When the cucumber is ready, transfer it to a chopping board and chop into brave chunks. Dress with the juice of the remaining lemon half.

Divide the watercress yoghurt between your serving plates and top with the kipper hash. Serve with the griddled and dressed cucumbers and finish with a pinch of the remaining watercress.

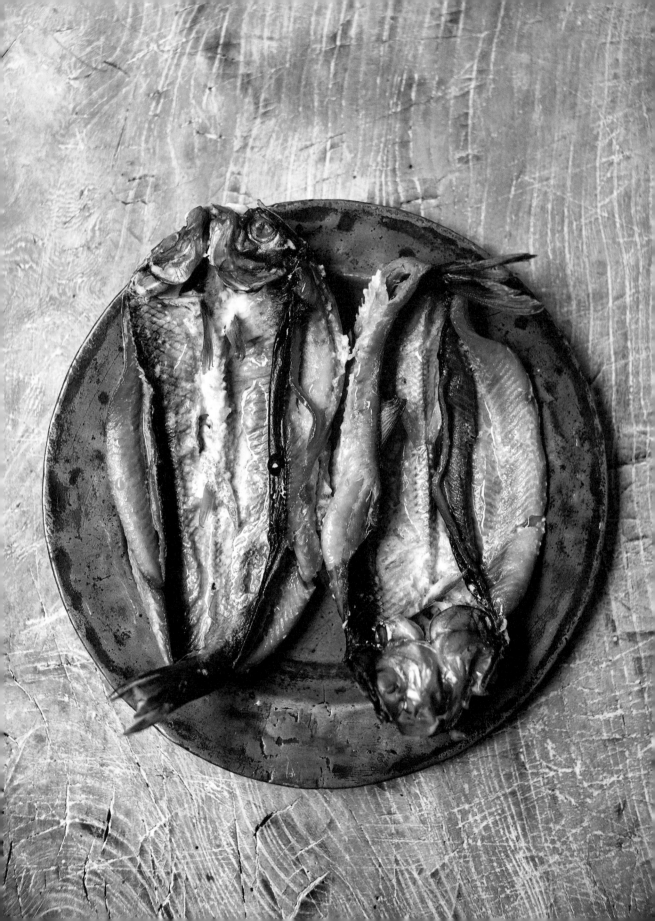

GIN-CURED SALMON WITH CREAMY SCRAMBLED EGGS

There's nothing quite like curing your own salmon at home, and it isn't difficult at all – all you need is time. A simple cure made from gin and citrus makes for a delicate but beautiful flavour, which works perfectly with creamy scrambled eggs.

SERVES 4

—

½ tablespoon coriander seeds

1 tablespoon peppercorns (*mixed, if possible*)

6 juniper berries

150g fine sea salt

125g caster sugar

50ml gin

1 lemon

400g salmon fillet, skin on and pin-boned

TO SERVE

—

10 large eggs

sea salt and freshly ground black pepper

½ a bunch of chives

4 slices of sourdough bread

50g butter

Start curing a whole day before you plan to serve the salmon.

Lightly toast the coriander seeds, peppercorns and juniper berries in a dry frying pan over a low heat for 1–2 minutes, then grind in a mortar and pestle (or a spice grinder) until you have a fine powder. Spoon into a bowl and add the sea salt, sugar and gin, then finely grate in the lemon zest. Stir everything together until well mixed, then spoon half the mixture into a tray not much bigger than the salmon fillet. Place the salmon in the tray, skin side down, and cover with the remaining salt mixture. Cover tightly with clingfilm and pop into the fridge for 12 hours. After the first 12 hours, turn the salmon over in the cure and spoon over any liquid that has formed at the bottom of the tray and any of the cure that has fallen off. Cover and return to the fridge for a further 12 hours or overnight.

When you want to serve your salmon, wash the cure off and pat the fish dry. Slice the salmon into thin slices, discarding the skin. Any remaining salmon can be stored, covered, in the fridge for up to a week.

When you are ready to serve, crack the eggs into a large bowl and season with salt and pepper. Finely slice the chives and add to the bowl, whisking everything together. Place a large non-stick frying pan on a medium heat and pop your sourdough into the toaster. Add half the butter to the pan, saving the rest for the toast. Pour your eggs into the pan and gently scramble, until just cooked and a little creamy still. Butter the toast, and serve topped with the creamy eggs, a few slices of the cured salmon and a wedge of lemon.

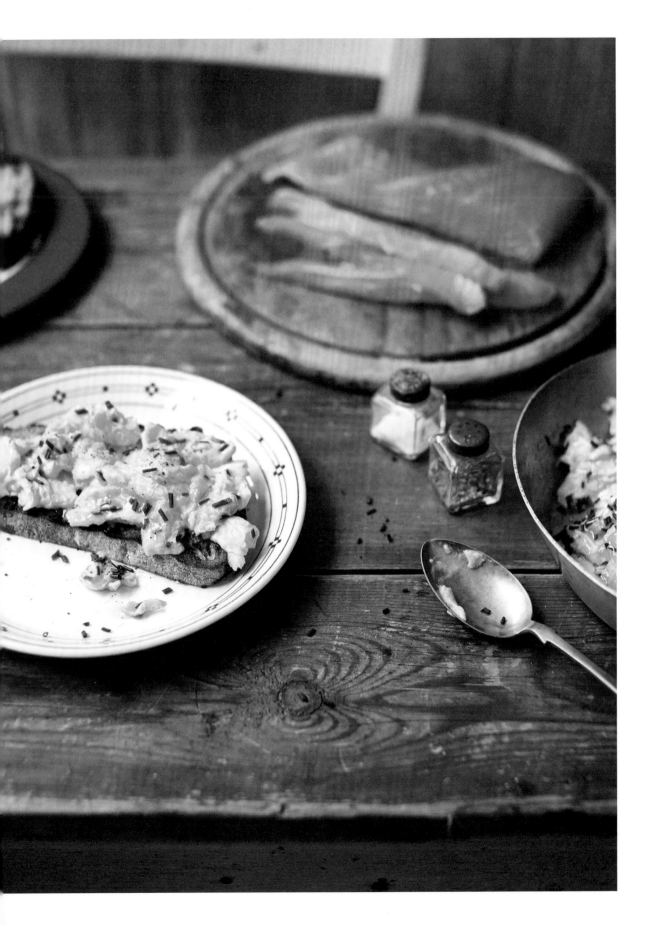

CHORIZO, TOMATO AND CHICKPEAS ON TOAST

I know it's not everyone's cup of tea, but I love beans on toast. It's probably mostly due to nostalgia, but I do think there is a place for them in life. Beans and pulses are nutrient-rich foods that we should be eating more of, and they make a fantastic breakfast. This recipe uses chickpeas for a twist on the classic and it can either be slow-cooked, using dried chickpeas, or a quicker affair using tinned. Either way it's a perfect dish for the weekend, and when made in bulk can be easily reheated during the week for a speedier meal.

SERVES 4

—

150g cooking chorizo *(a whole sausage, not the sliced kind)*

450g ripe vine tomatoes

3 garlic cloves

1 bunch of flat-leaf parsley

extra virgin olive oil

50ml sherry *(oloroso works well)*

1 tablespoon tomato purée

300g dried chickpeas, cooked, or 2 x 400g tins of chickpeas, drained

sea salt and freshly ground black pepper

a splash of sherry vinegar

4 slices of sourdough, or your favourite bread

Chop the chorizo and tomatoes into small pieces of about 1cm, and peel and finely chop 2 of the garlic cloves. Finely chop the parsley stalks and chop the leaves, keeping them separate.

Place a large non-stick frying pan on a medium heat and pour in a glug of olive oil. Fry the chorizo for a couple of minutes, then add the sherry. Bring it to the boil, then let it cook away. Continue to cook the chorizo for around 5 minutes, stirring often, until golden. Reduce the heat a little and spoon out any excess oil – you only need to leave a tablespoon in the pan.

Add the chopped garlic, fry for a minute, then stir in the tomato purée. Fry for a further 1–2 minutes, then add the chopped tomatoes, chickpeas and 200ml of water. Gently bring to the boil, season well, then reduce the heat to a simmer and cover the pan with the lid. Cook for 20 minutes, then remove the lid, turn the heat up a little and cook for a further 10–15 minutes uncovered. You should end up with a thick, rich sauce. If it still looks a little watery, continue to cook uncovered and turn the heat up a little. Finish with a splash of sherry vinegar and stir in the chopped parsley.

Toast the sourdough, then cut the remaining garlic clove in half and rub the top side of the toast with the cut side of the garlic. Drizzle with a little extra virgin olive oil and spoon over the chorizo chickpeas. Serve straight away.

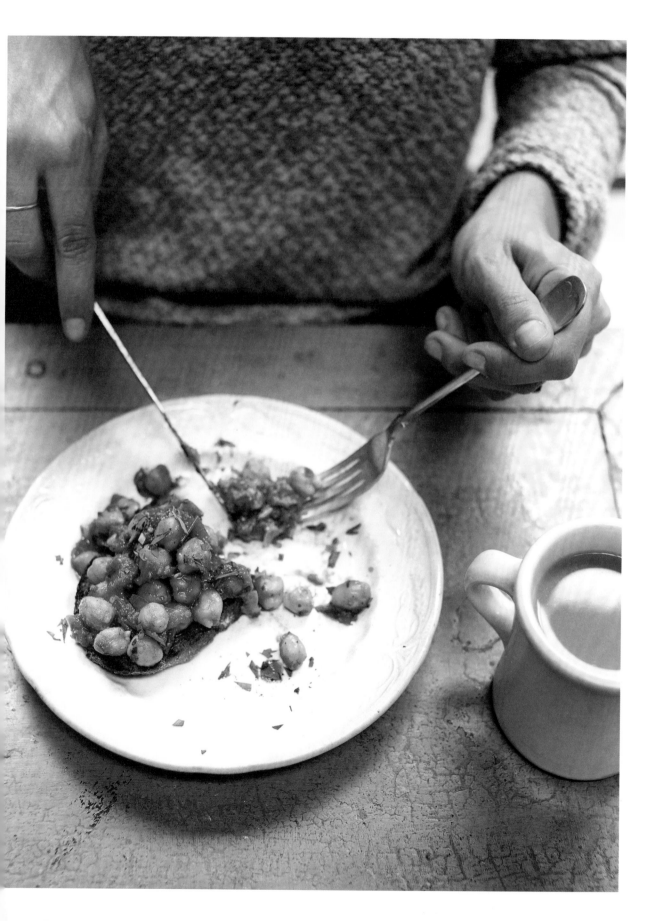

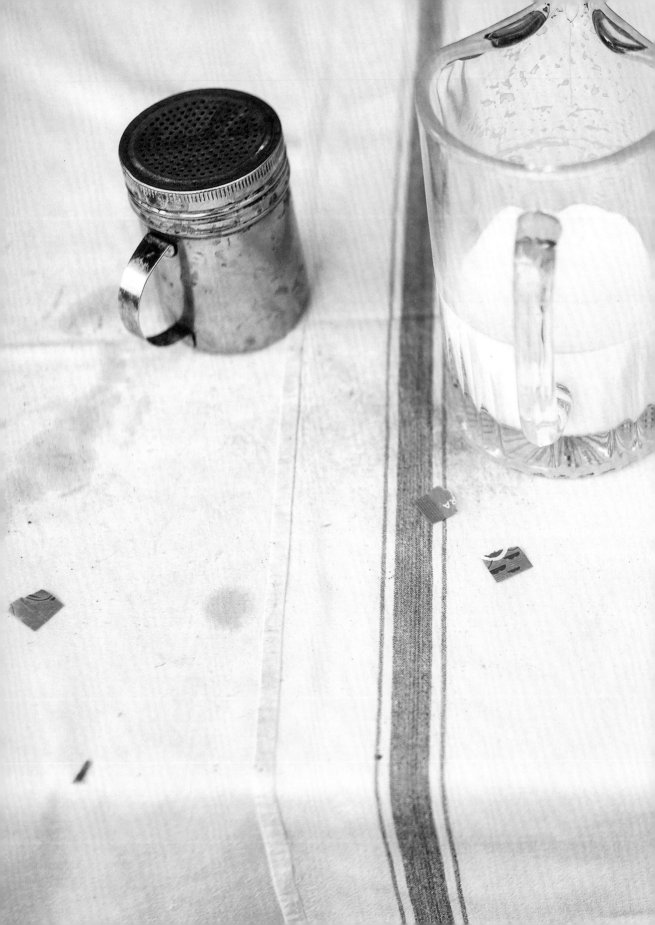

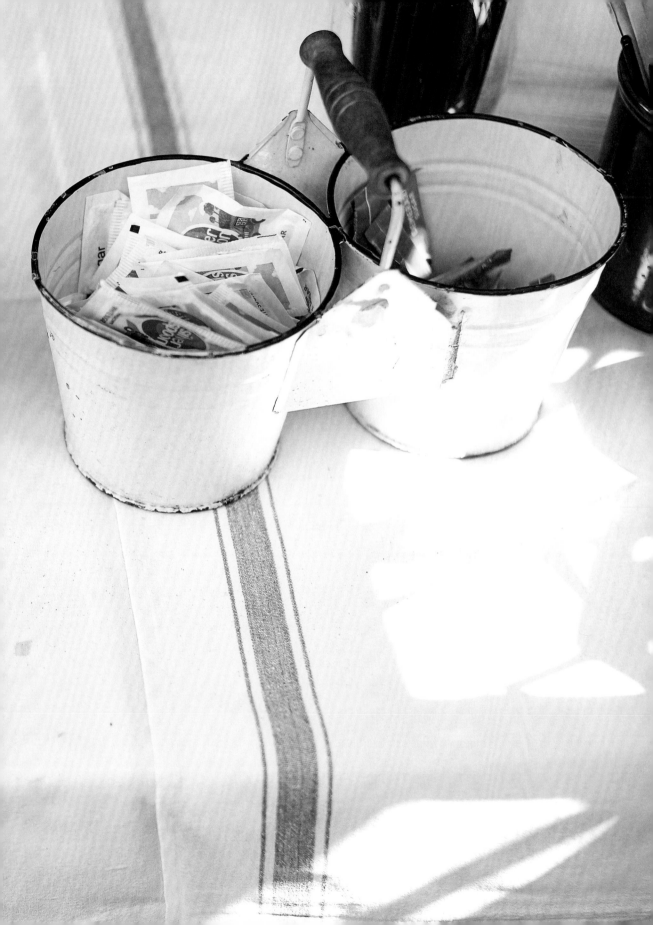

REFRIED LENTILS WITH CRISPY SAUSAGE, PEPPER SALSA AND AVOCADO

I have Pete to thank for this corker of a recipe; having always been a fan of refried beans, he asked me what would happen if we used lentils instead. So we did and it's utterly delicious! And nutritious too – lentils are a great way to start the day, as they will keep you feeling full for ages. It works best if you cook the lentils ahead and fry at the last minute, but if you don't have time don't worry, it'll still be great. Feel free to top it with a poached egg for something a little heartier. And for a veggie alternative just leave out the sausage.

SERVES 4
—

2 red onions

½ a bunch of coriander

1 jalapeño chill

½ teaspoon coriander seeds

olive oil

300g dried brown lentils

2 red peppers

1 dried chipotle chilli

2 garlic cloves

½ teaspoon smoked paprika

300g ripe vine tomatoes

1 tablespoon red wine vinegar

4 good-quality sausages

2 avocados

2 limes

60g wild rocket

Put a large kettle on to boil. Peel and finely chop the onions. Pick the coriander leaves, keep to one side and finely chop the stalks. Finely chop the Jalapeño and crush the coriander seeds in a mortar and pestle. Place a large non-stick saucepan over a medium heat and pour in a drizzle of olive oil. Add the onions, coriander stalks and jalapeño and sauté for 10 minutes, until softened but not coloured. Stir in the coriander seeds, fry for a couple more minutes, then add the lentils. Stir in 800ml of boiling water and bring back to the boil. Season well, then reduce the heat, pop on the lid and simmer for 40 minutes, until the lentils are cooked and beginning to break down.

Meanwhile, blacken the peppers by either placing them directly on a gas flame, or griddling them in a griddle pan, turning regularly until blackened all over. Pop them into a bowl, cover with clingfilm and let stand for around 5 minutes. By then the pepper skins should flake away easily. Remove the skins, stalks, and seeds. Slice the flesh into thin strips and leave to one side.

Place the chipotle chilli in a small bowl and pour in just enough boiling water to cover. After a few minutes, it should have softened; carefully remove from the bowl and finely chop.

Peel and finely chop the garlic and chop the tomatoes. Place a medium-size pan over a medium heat and pour in a glug of olive oil. Add the garlic and chipotle chilli and fry for 1 minute, then add the peppers and paprika. Fry for a few more minutes, then add the tomatoes. Season well and gradually bring everything to a simmer, then leave to bubble away gently for 10 minutes, until you have a thick and rich tomato sauce, adding a splash of water if it gets too thick. Add the splash of red wine vinegar and set aside. When it's cooled down a bit, chop the coriander leaves, then stir through.

While the salsa is ticking away, place a large frying pan on a medium heat and add a drizzle of olive oil. Squeeze the sausage meat out of its skins and break it up into the frying pan. Fry for 5–10 minutes, until cooked through and crisp all over.

When your lentils are cooked, roughly purée them with a stick blender. Spoon the lentils into the pan with the sausage meat and fry for about 15 minutes, stirring occasionally, so you end up with crispy fried lentils.

While they are frying, peel, destone and slice the avocados, and roughly chop the rocket and dress with the juice of 1 lime. Cut the remaining lime into quarters.

Serve the refried lentils with a dollop of the red pepper salsa, the dressed avocado and rocket and a wedge of lime on the side.

ROAST SWEET POTATO, PANCETTA AND MAPLE LOAF

This recipe started life as part of a sugar-free feature I wrote. It won everyone over and has been a firm favourite ever since. I have now tweaked it slightly and I do use maple syrup in it – however, if you are avoiding sugar you can absolutely leave it out. I guarantee you it will still be delicious. Once the loaf has cooled it freezes really well, so make it, eat what you like and freeze the rest for a rainy day. Very virtuous.

SERVES 10

—

500g sweet potatoes

1 teaspoon ground cinnamon

1 teaspoon mixed spice

½ teaspoon sea salt

125ml olive oil, plus extra for drizzling

1 orange

6 rashers of pancetta *(if you are veggie, the loaf is just as delicious without)*

2 large eggs

50g natural yoghurt

50g pecans

3 tablespoons maple syrup

200g wholemeal or plain flour

2 teaspoons bicarbonate of soda

Preheat the oven to 170°C/gas 3. Grease a 1 litre loaf tin and line with greaseproof paper.

Peel and chop the sweet potatoes into 2–3cm chunks and pop them into a large roasting tray. Sprinkle over the cinnamon, mixed spice, sea salt and a good glug of olive oil. Finely grate over the orange zest, halve the orange and squeeze over the juice. Toss everything together and put into the oven for 25 minutes. Then drape the pancetta slices over the sweet potato and pop back into the oven for a further 10 minutes, until the sweet potato is golden and cooked through and the pancetta is crisp. Remove from the oven (but leave the oven on) and set aside to cool a little.

Push the cooked pancetta to one side of the tray, then spoon the sweet potato into a food processor and blitz to a purée. Add the eggs, yoghurt, most of the pecans, the maple syrup, flour, bicarbonate of soda and the 125ml olive oil, and blitz again until just combined. Crumble in the pancetta and fold through. Using a spatula, scrape the mixture into the lined loaf tin and then chop and sprinkle over the remaining pecans. Pop the tin into the preheated oven for 1 hour, then check with a skewer. It should come out clean. If not, return the loaf to the oven for a further 10 minutes, until golden and cooked through.

Leave to cool in the tin for 5 minutes before cooling completely on a rack. Serve straight up or toasted. It is delicious with butter beaten with a little maple syrup.

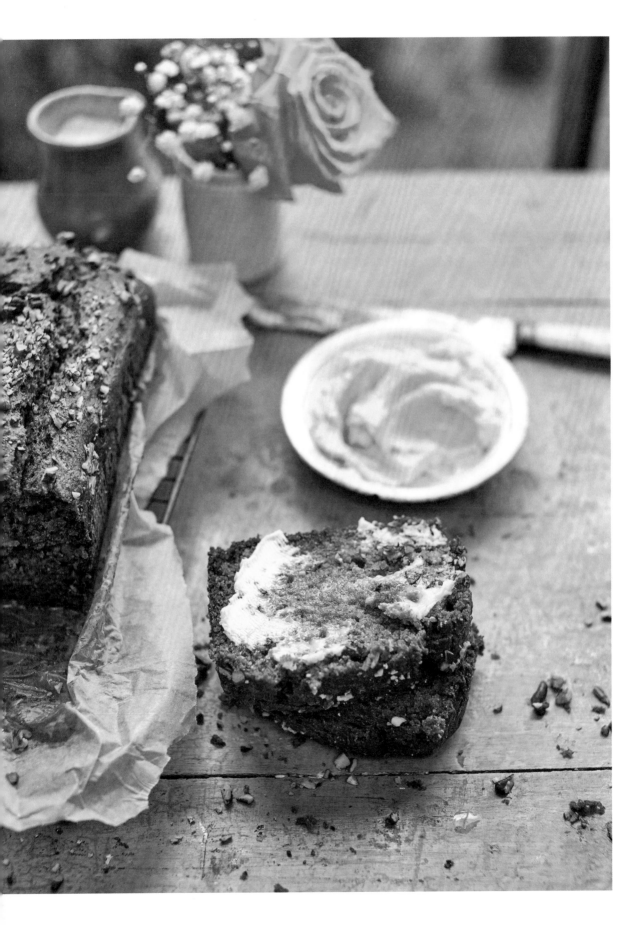

COURGETTE, COCONUT AND CARDAMOM LOAF WITH HONEY BUTTER

There is something terribly Mediterranean about a slice of chocolate marble cake and a glass of milk for breakfast, which was our morning meal of choice growing up! However, we've come a long way since then, and I genuinely want something better for myself most mornings. So this is my twist on our teenage years; instead of chocolate cake it's a dense and delicious courgette and coconut loaf, laced with crushed cardamom and served with honey-sweetened yoghurt. Delicious.

SERVES 8-10
—

125g unsalted butter, plus extra for greasing

8 green cardamom pods

2 small courgettes *(about 250g)*

175ml olive oil

125g golden caster sugar

2 large eggs

1 lime

a pinch of salt

60g unsweetened desiccated coconut

325g wholemeal or normal self-raising flour

¼ teaspoon bicarbonate of soda

3 tablespoons honey

NB If you can't get unsweetened desiccated coconut, buy the sweetened stuff and soak it in boiling water for a couple of minutes, then drain.

Preheat the oven to 170°C/gas 3. Grease a 1 litre loaf tin with a little butter, then line with greaseproof paper.

Gently crush the cardamom pods in a pestle and mortar, then discard the outsides and finely grind the black seeds, Coarsely grate the courgettes and leave to one side.

In a large mixing bowl whisk together the oil and sugar, then beat in the eggs. Fold in the ground cardamom seeds, grated courgette and finely grate in the lime zest. Add a pinch of salt and stir in the coconut. Add the flour and bicarbonate of soda and fold everything together until just combined. Pour the mixture into the lined tin and bake in the middle of the oven for 1 hour and 15 minutes. When the time is up, check the loaf – it may need up to 10–15 minutes longer. It's ready when a skewer inserted into the centre comes out clean. Remove from the oven and leave to cool in the tin for 10 minutes before transferring to a cooling rack.

While the loaf is baking make the honey butter. Beat the butter and honey together in a mixing bowl with a wooden spoon, or in a free standing mixer, until pale and creamy. Mix in a good pinch of salt and spoon into a serving bowl, if using straight away, or roll it into a log in greaseproof and pop it in the fridge until needed.

Serve the courgette loaf cut in slices, either fresh or lightly grilled, with the honey butter on the side.

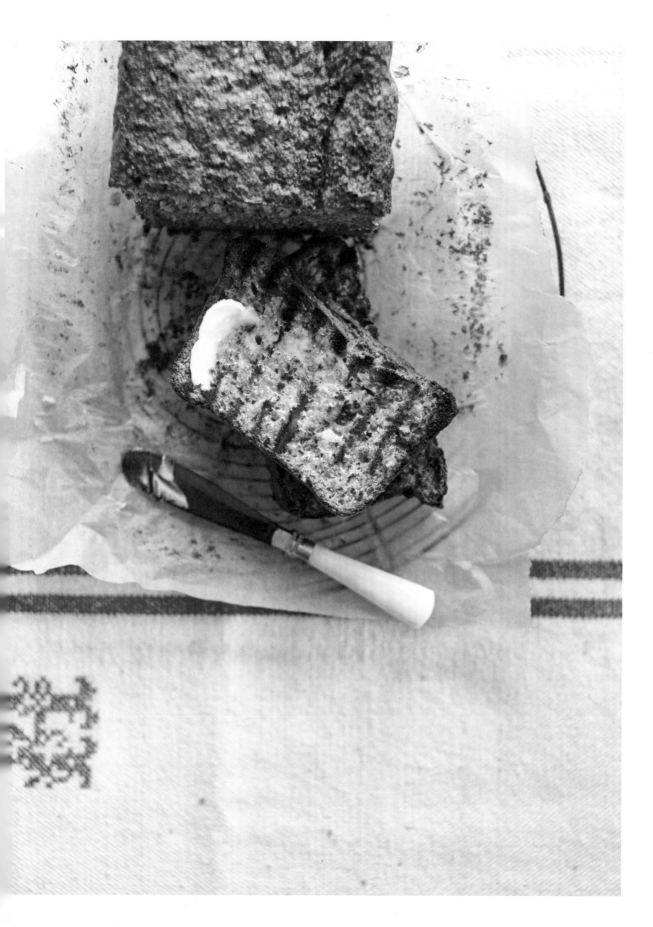

BREAKFAST ON THE RUN

Sometimes, despite all our best efforts and intentions, there just really isn't time for a sit-down breakfast. Here are three of my 'go-to' smoothies – they taste delicious and will keep you going when you're on the run.

THE CLASSIC

—

1 medjool date

1 heaped tablespoon rolled oats

a good pinch of ground cinnamon

1 small banana, chopped and frozen

1 tablespoon bran

250ml full-fat cow's milk or almond milk *(or any milk of your choice – hazelnut or coconut milk work well too)*

a drizzle of honey *(I only use honey if I am using cow's milk, as the nut milks tend to have a natural sweetness to them already)*

Remove the stone from the date and discard. Place all the ingredients in a blender and leave to sit for a couple of minutes. Blitz for a minute, until you have a smooth and creamy texture, adding a splash more milk if it's a little on the thick side. Serve immediately.

RASPBERRY MILKSHAKE

—

1 small banana, chopped and frozen

1 heaped tablespoon rolled oats

a handful of raspberries

8 grapes *(or just a few more raspberries)*

1 large tablespoon organic black cherry yoghurt *(also delicious with dairy-free coconut yoghurt)*

250ml freshly pressed apple juice

Place all the ingredients in a blender and leave to sit for a couple of minutes. Blitz until you have a smooth and creamy smoothie, adding a splash more apple juice if it is a little thick. Blitz again, then serve.

THE POPEYE

—

a sprig of mint

1 small banana, chopped and frozen

a handful of blueberries

a large handful of baby leaf spinach

a squeeze of lime juice

1 tablespoon milled flax seed

250ml freshly pressed apple juice

Pick the mint leaves and discard the stalk. Pop everything into a blender and leave to sit for a couple of minutes. Blitz for a minute, until you have a super-smooth texture. Add a splash more apple juice if it's a little thick, then blitz again and serve straight away.

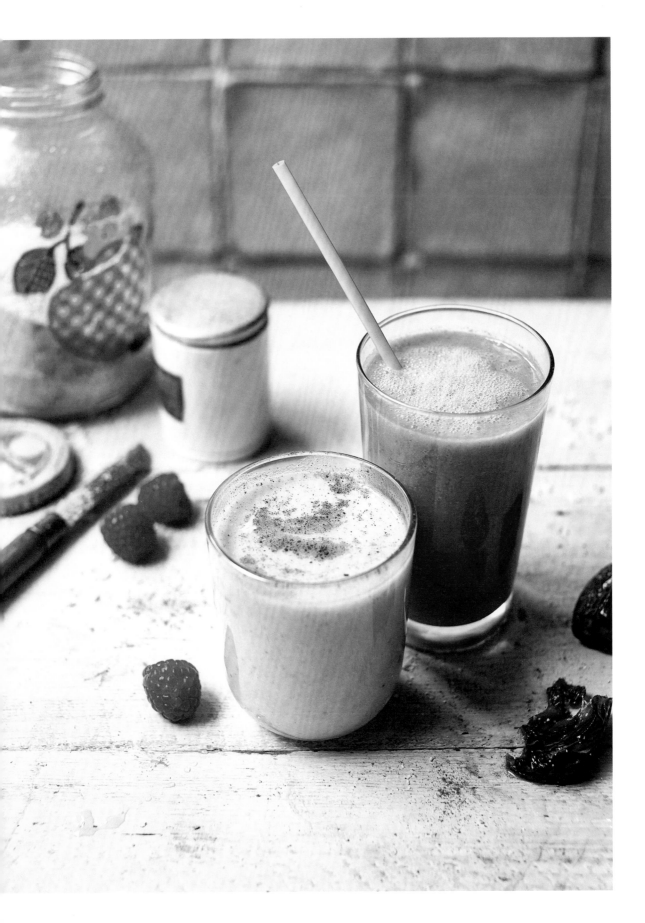

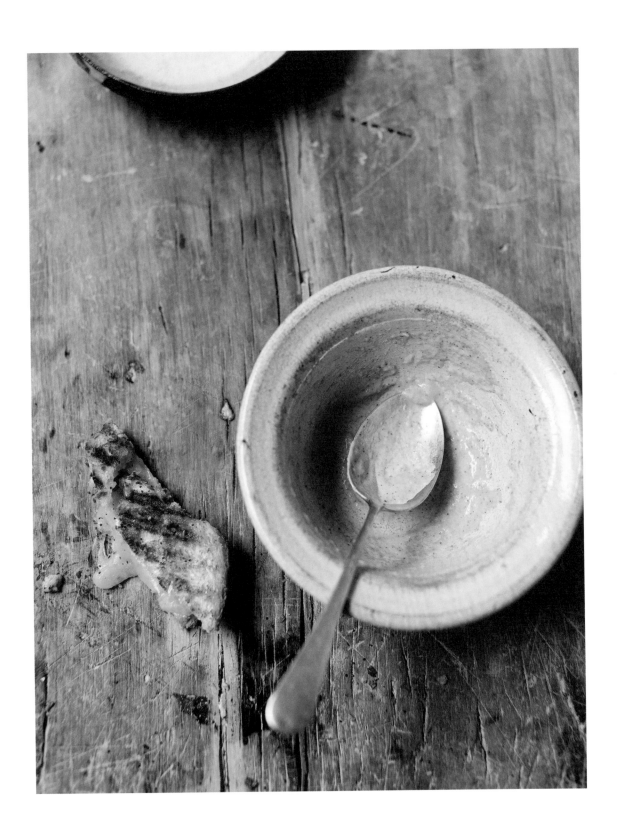

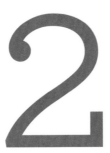

BOWL FOOD

—

I was once asked what my favourite comfort food was and I knew the answer straight away: anything I can eat from a bowl with a spoon. If I can eat it from my favourite bowl, with only one piece of cutlery, the chances are I will find it comforting. Soup is the most obvious contender, and although there really are many others (curry, noodles, pasta and mashed potato all spring to mind), soup is a firm favourite for many reasons.

It's warming, literally, and it reminds me of being young and being looked after. Even now, if I know someone is poorly or needs comforting I make them soup; it's the ultimate uncomplicated meal. So this chapter is a big up to all soups – my perfect 'meal in a bowl'.

ZUPPA DI FARRO WITH ROSEMARY AND PINE NUT OIL

This soup was my food highlight when filming in Tuscany many years ago; I stopped for lunch at a small workman's-style café and just copied what the locals ate. It looked unassuming but I knew it had to be good, and I wasn't disappointed. This is my homage to that heavenly bowl.

SERVES 6
—

200g dried borlotti beans

2 onions

4 garlic cloves

2 carrots

2 sticks of celery

½ a bunch of rosemary

150g guanciale or pancetta

olive oil

2 ripe tomatoes

a few sprigs of thyme and parsley

175g farro

sea salt and freshly ground black
    pepper

50g pine nuts

Rinse the beans and discard any old-looking ones. Place in a large bowl with plenty of cold water, so they're covered by at least 5cm. Leave to soak for 12 hours or overnight.

When you are ready to make your soup, start by preparing the base. Peel and finely chop the onions, garlic and carrots. Trim and finely chop the celery. Pick the rosemary leaves and finely chop. Cut the guanciale or pancetta into small cubes.

Place a large saucepan on a medium-low heat and pour in a good few glugs of olive oil. Add all the chopped veg, the guanciale and half the rosemary and sauté for 12–15 minutes, until soft and sticky. Finely chop the tomatoes and add to the pan, along with the drained beans and 2.5 litres of water. Tie the thyme and parsley together with butcher's string and add to the pot. Gently bring to the boil, skim off any scum that comes to the surface, then reduce the heat to the lowest setting. Cover with a lid, leaving it just ajar, and leave to tick away for 3 hours, until the beans are soft and tender. Check the water occasionally and add more if it reduces too much.

After 3 hours, gently mash the cooked beans with a potato masher, breaking some of them down, then add the farro to the pot. Season generously and bring back to the boil. Reduce to simmer again, and cook for a further hour.

While the farro is cooking, make the rosemary and pine nut oil. Place a small frying pan on a medium-low heat and scatter in the pine nuts. Toast until golden, then add the rest of the chopped rosemary and 6 tablespoons of olive oil. Heat for 4–5 minutes, or until the rosemary starts to sizzle. Remove from the heat and leave to one side. When the soup is ready, discard the herb bunch, check the seasoning, and ladle into your bowls. Finish with the crispy rosemary and pine nut oil. Absolutely delicious.

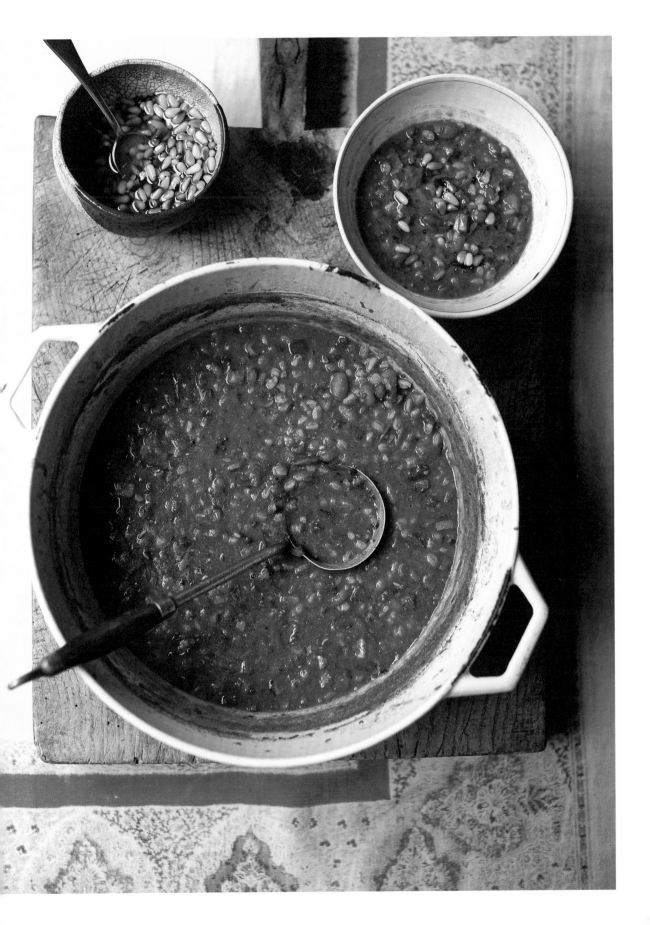

CHILLED AVOCADO SOUP WITH GINGER SESAME RADISHES

A quick and easy soup that is full of goodness. Avocado is a top source of unsaturated fat, which is great for your heart, reducing the risk of heart disease - and you won't feel like you're being short-changed on flavour.

SERVES 4

—

½ red chilli

½ a garlic clove

a 2cm piece of ginger

½ tablespoon toasted sesame
   seeds

1 tablespoon sesame oil

1 tablespoon low-salt soy sauce

¼ of a cucumber

4 radishes

2 limes

2 ripe avocados

½ a bunch of coriander

600ml ice-cold water

12 ice cubes

a few pinches of basil cress,
   optional

sea salt and freshly ground black
   pepper

Start by preparing the garnish. Deseed and finely slice the chilli, peel and finely grate the garlic and the ginger. Place in a bowl with the sesame seeds, sesame oil and soy sauce. Cut the cucumber in half lengthways and scoop out the seeds. Finely slice into half-moons and add to the bowl. Trim and roughly chop the radishes and bash lightly in a mortar and pestle to break them up a little, then add to the bowl and toss everything together. Squeeze in the juice of half a lime, stir through and leave to one side.

Halve the avocados, remove the stones and scoop the flesh into a liquidiser. Pick the coriander leaves and add most of them to the liquidiser with the remaining lime juice, and pour in the ice-cold water. Season generously and blitz until you have a creamy smooth soup, adding a splash more water if it is very thick.

Pour the avocado soup into 4 bowls and stir 3 ice cubes into each (don't worry if the soup is a little thick, you want the ice cubes to melt slightly to thin it out and chill it at the same time). After a couple of minutes, garnish with the dressed veg, and finish with the cress and remaining coriander leaves. Serve straight away.

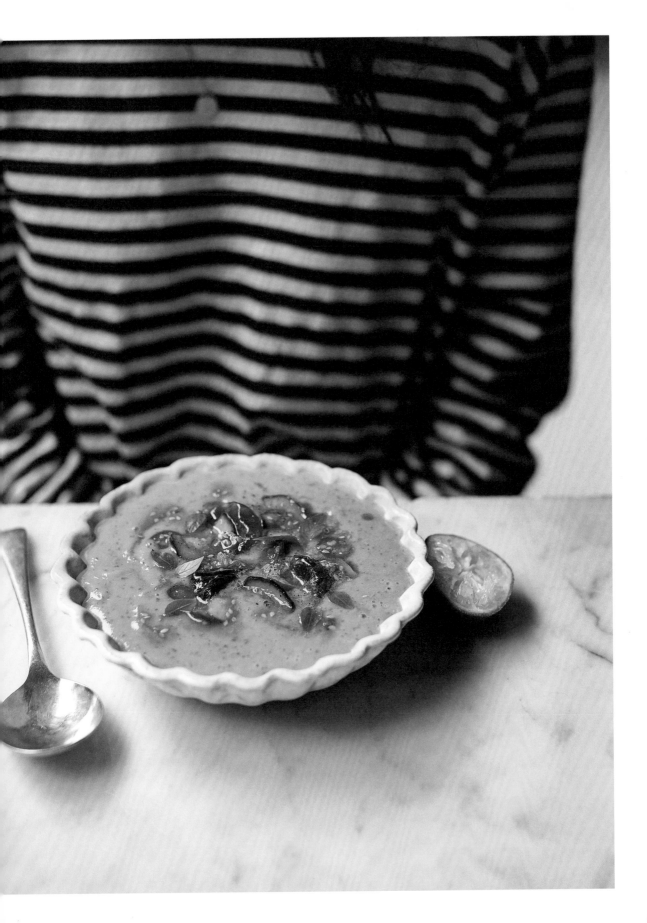

PARSNIP, MUSTARD AND COMTÉ SOUP

When we were growing up, my poor yiayia would slave away for hours over a traditional Cypriot soup that contained little cubes of halloumi, only to find that we'd sit there and just pick out the cheese. I used to love finding little pools of treasure in my soup! (I wasn't a fan of the soup itself, I'm afraid.) And I still do – it suddenly makes a simple week-night meal feel a little more substantial and special. This one is a particular favourite – the combination of flavours works perfectly and I just can't get enough of the slightly molten Comté.

SERVES 4

—

1 onion

1 apple

1 stick of celery

olive oil

750g parsnips

100g Comté or Gruyère

½ a bunch of sage

1 tablespoon English mustard

1 litre vegetable stock

300ml full-fat milk

1 tablespoon English mustard

sea salt and freshly ground black pepper

a large knob of butter

Trim and peel the onion, and finely chop. Halve the apple, remove the core, and chop. Trim and finely chop the celery. Place a large saucepan on a medium-low heat and drizzle in a little olive oil. Add the chopped veg (including the apple) and sauté gently for 12–15 minutes, until soft and sticky but not coloured.

Meanwhile peel the parsnips and cut into 2-3cm pieces. Cut the cheese into 1cm cubes, and pick the sage leaves.

When the veg in the pan are ready, stir in the mustard and fry for a minute, then add the chopped parsnips and the vegetable stock and gently bring to the boil. Reduce the heat to a simmer and leave to gently bubble away for 15 minutes, or until the parsnips are cooked through and tender. Remove the pan from the heat and stir in the milk. Using a stick blender, blitz the soup until smooth, then season to taste. If it is a little thick, just add a splash more milk. Return the pan to a low heat to keep warm.

When the soup is ready, place a small frying pan on a medium-low heat and add the butter with just a drizzle of olive oil. When the butter has melted, add the picked sage leaves and fry just until they are crisp.

Divide the cheese between the bowls and ladle the hot soup on top. Garnish with a few crispy sage leaves and a drizzle of the flavoured butter.

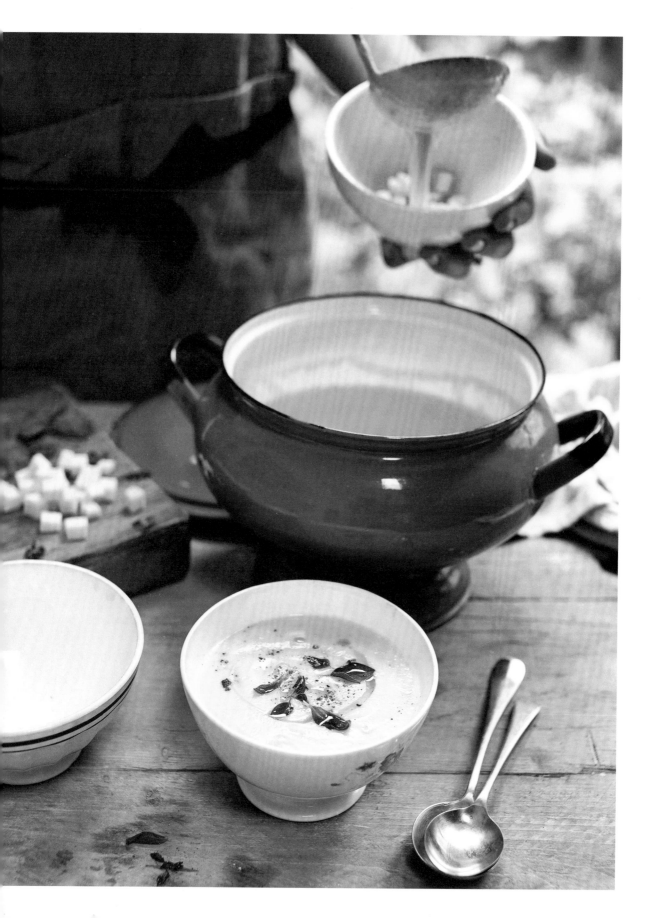

PETE'S BROCCOLI SOUP WITH STILTON SOLDIERS

If I had to pick one soup to eat for the rest of my life it would be this one. It's not mind-alteringly unique, but it is familiar, homely and just a beautiful celebration of my favourite vegetable. Also, it's the first thing Pete ever made me, years before we got together. Followed by a fish-finger sarnie and jelly and ice cream. All my favourite things. He even saved a cube of undiluted jelly for me, just like my mum used to. I should've known then really that I was going to marry him. (Although the Stilton soldiers are all me; Pete hates blue cheese – it's upsetting.)

SERVES 6

—

1 onion

2 garlic cloves

2 leeks

50g butter

olive oil

10 sprigs of thyme

600g broccoli

1 medium potato *(approx 150g)*

1 litre vegetable stock

100g Cheddar

75g Stilton

6 slices of good-quality bloomer

runny honey

200ml single cream

sea salt and freshly ground black
   pepper

Peel the onion and garlic and chop finely. Trim the leeks, slice finely, then wash in a colander to remove any dirt. Place a large saucepan on a medium-low heat, add a little butter, a drizzle of olive oil and the chopped and sliced veg. Pick the thyme leaves and add to the pan, then sauté gently for 15 minutes, until soft and sticky but not coloured.

Trim the broccoli and cut into even-sized florets, slicing the stalk too. Peel the potato and cut into small even-size chunks. Add the veg to the pan and pour in the vegetable stock. Turn up the heat and bring to the boil. As soon as it start to bubble, reduce the heat, cover with a lid and simmer for 12–15 minutes, or until the broccoli and potato are tender.

While the soup is cooking, get your soldiers ready. Place a griddle pan or a large non-stick frying pan on a high heat. Coarsely grate the Cheddar, slice or crumble up the Stilton, and mix them together. Butter the 6 bread slices lightly on both sides and divide the cheese between 3 of the slices. Put the remaining bread on top, then griddle or fry the sandwiches. If using a frying pan, try placing something on top of the sandwiches to act as a weight and push them into the pan. Turn them over when charred or golden and continue with the second side. When they are ready, transfer to a chopping board and drizzle with a little honey.

When the soup is ready, blitz with a hand blender until completely smooth. Pour in the cream, blitz again, and season to taste. Slice the toasties into soldiers and serve alongside bowls of the hot soup. Heavenly.

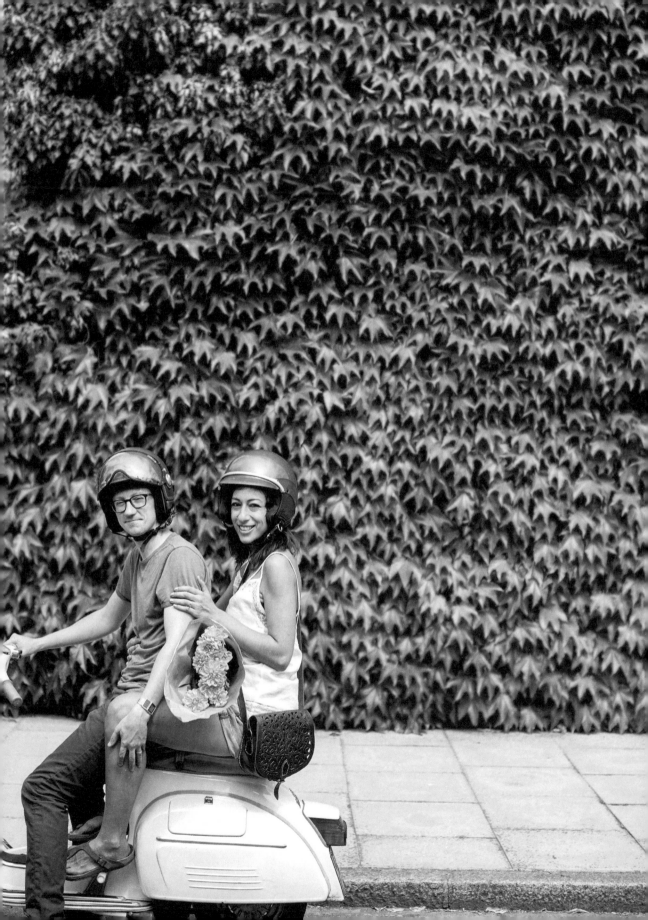

ROAST SWEET POTATO, SPINACH AND CHICKPEA SOUP

I initially wrote this recipe for my parents, trying to recreate a soup they had on holiday (I was given a list of the key ingredients), and it has become a firm family favourite. A little bit smooth and a little bit chunky, this is a rich and wholesome soup.

SERVES 6

—

550g sweet potatoes (approx. 3)

olive oil

1 x 400g tin of chickpeas

sea salt and freshly ground black pepper

1 lemon

1½ teaspoons ground cumin

2 onions

2 garlic cloves

½ a bunch of coriander

1 green chilli

1 teaspoon ground coriander

800ml vegetable stock

1 x 400ml tin of reduced-fat coconut milk

200g spinach

Preheat your oven to 200°C/gas 6. Rub the sweet potatoes with a little oil and place on a large roasting tray. Pop into the oven and roast for 30 minutes, until almost cooked.

Drain the chickpeas, and when the potatoes have had half an hour in the oven, scatter them around the tray. Drizzle with a little oil, season generously, finely grate over the lemon zest and sprinkle with ½ teaspoon of ground cumin. Toss everything together and pop into the oven for a further 15 minutes, until the chickpeas are golden and crispy and the potatoes are cooked through.

While the tray is in the oven, start the base. Place a large non-stick saucepan on a medium-low heat and add a glug of olive oil. Peel and finely chop the onions and the garlic and sauté for around 10 minutes, until soft. Pick the coriander leaves and keep to one side, and finely chop the stalks. Halve, deseed and finely slice the chilli, then add it to the pan with the coriander stalks, the remaining teaspoon of ground cumin and the ground coriander and fry for a further 3–4 minutes.

Carefully, roughly chop the sweet potato and add it to the pan. Add most of the chickpeas, reserving some for garnish, and pour in the stock and coconut milk. Gently bring everything to the boil, season well, then reduce to a simmer and cover. Cook for around 10 minutes.

When the soup is ready, add the spinach and cook for a couple more minutes. Remove the pan from the heat, add most of the coriander leaves and blitz the soup until smooth, using a stick blender. If it's a little on the thick side, add a bit more stock or water until you get to the texture and thickness that you like. Squeeze in the lemon juice and stir through. Taste and adjust the seasoning, then serve sprinkled with the remaining crispy chickpeas and any remaining coriander leaves.

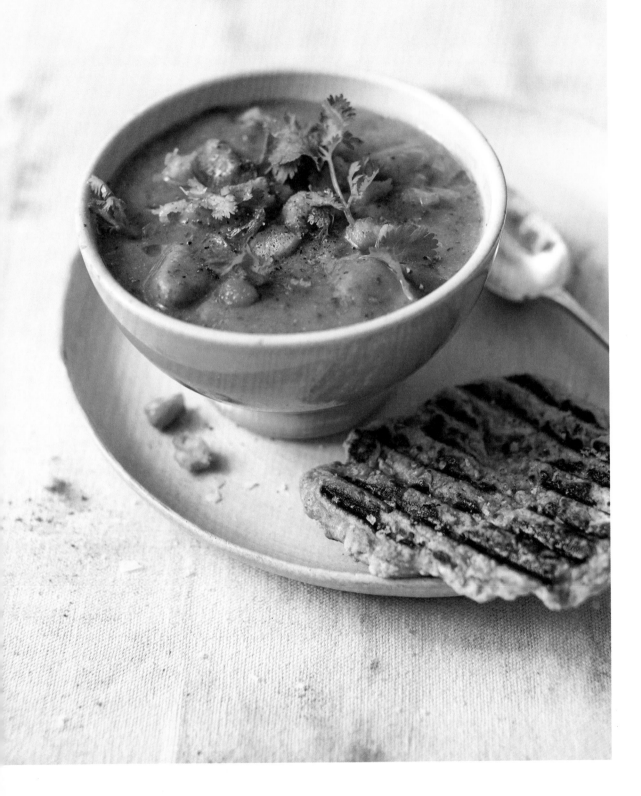

ROASTED CAULIFLOWER AND COCONUT SOUP

We adore this soup at home and make it often after work, when we are a little tired and just want to curl up with a bowl of something warming. It's easy to do, doesn't need much attention, and is rich, lightly spiced and deliciously creamy.

SERVES 4-6
—

2 onions

600g cauliflower

4 garlic cloves

1 heaped teaspoon ground cinnamon

1 heaped teaspoon ras el hanout

sea salt and freshly ground black pepper

olive oil

a handful of unsweetened coconut flakes

1 x 400ml tin of reduced-fat coconut milk

600ml vegetable stock

2-3 tablespoons chilli oil

Preheat your oven to 180°C/gas 4.

Peel and cut the onions into 1cm wedges and trim then cut the cauliflower into even-sized florets. If it has the leaves on, don't cut them off, roast those too. Place it all in a roasting tray with the unpeeled garlic cloves and sprinkle with the cinnamon and ras el hanout. Season well, and drizzle everything with a good glug of olive oil. Toss it all together and pop into the oven for 25–30 minutes, until cooked through and a little charred. Scatter the coconut flakes on to a small tray and pop into the oven for the last few minutes to toast – they should only need 3-4 minutes.

When the veg are ready, remove the garlic cloves and scrape all the veg into a large saucepan. Squeeze the garlic out of its skins and add them too. Pour in the coconut milk, add the stock and gently bring to the boil. Reduce the heat a little and simmer for 5 minutes, then remove from the heat. Using a stick blender, blitz the soup until creamy and smooth, adding a splash more water if it is too thick.

Taste and adjust the seasoning, and serve topped with the toasted coconut flakes and a drizzle of chilli oil.

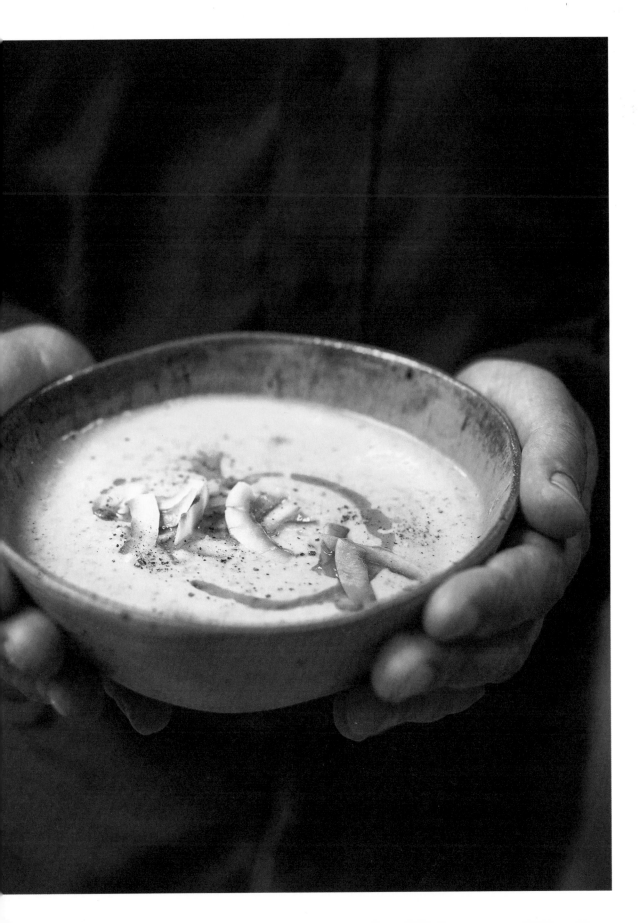

SALMOREJO

Not unlike the much-loved gazpacho, salmorejo is its simpler yet classier big sister. I love that by using only a few store cupboard ingredients you can quickly create something so delicious and refreshing – a glass of this on a hot summer's day is pure bliss. But please, please only make this with ripe, in-season tomatoes – this is not a winter soup and is easily ruined otherwise. You'll end up with bland mush.

SERVES 4

—

2 large hen's eggs or 4 quail's eggs

1 slice of serrano ham, 1cm thick

a few sprigs of flat-leaf parsley

8 large ripe tomatoes

1 garlic clove

2 thick slices of good white bread (*around 100g in total*)

125ml extra virgin olive oil

a splash of sherry vinegar

sea salt and freshly ground black pepper

8 ice cubes, to serve

Start by boiling your eggs. I boil hen's eggs for 7 minutes so they are hard-boiled, and quail's eggs for 3 minutes. Run them under cold running water, then peel and chop into bite-size pieces. Chop the serrano ham to a similar size. Pick and chop the parsley leaves.

Bring a large pan of water to the boil, then remove from the heat. Score a little cross on the top of each tomato, through the stalk, then plunge them into the boiling water for a minute or two, until you start to see the skin peeling away. Drain, then carefully peel off the tomato skins and discard.

Roughly chop the tomatoes and pop them into a blender. Peel and roughly chop the garlic and add it too, then blitz until completely smooth. Tear out the centre of the bread, discarding the crusts, then add to the blender and blitz until creamy. Finish by blitzing in the oil and a generous splash of vinegar. Season to taste, and add a little more vinegar if needed. Pour the salmorejo into a jug and pop into the fridge to chill for at least a couple of hours. Serve over ice, garnished with the chopped egg, serrano ham and some parsley.

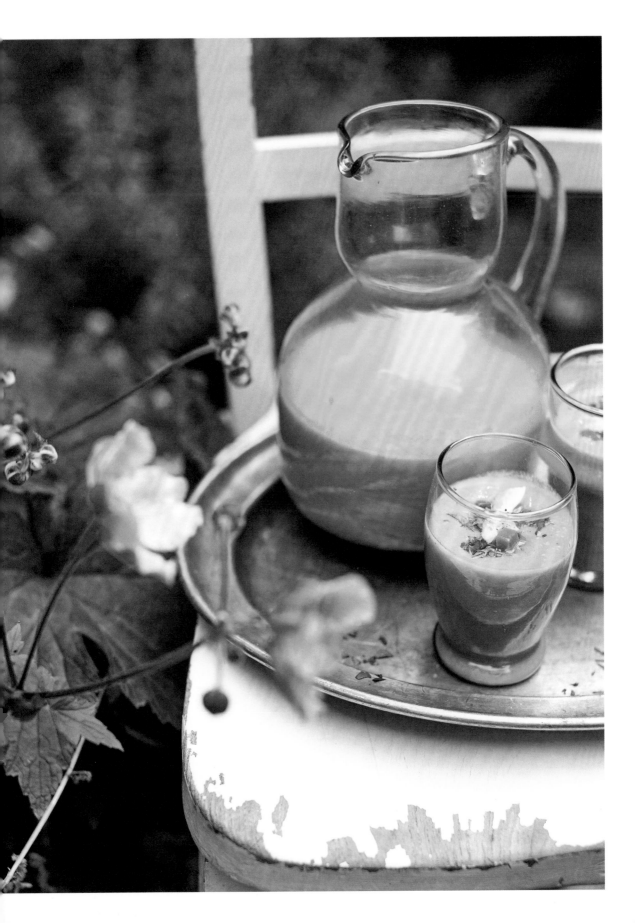

BREAD, LEEK AND CABBAGE LAYER SOUP

This my take on an Italian classic, a fantastic oven-baked soup made up of layers of stale bread, cheese and greens. It's wonderfully comforting and something a little different.

SERVES 6
—

800g Savoy cabbage or cavolo nero, or a mixture

4 leeks

2 onions

4 garlic cloves

1 large fennel bulb

200g mature Cheddar

½ a teaspoon fennel seeds

3 litres vegetable stock

½ a lemon

olive oil

½ a bunch of sage

4 anchovy fillets in oil

sea salt and freshly ground black pepper

1 large country-style loaf, ideally a few days old

Remove the stems from the cabbage and/or cavolo nero leaves and rinse well. Roll the leaves up like large cigars and cut into ½cm slices. Trim the leeks, slice to a similar thickness and rinse away any dirt. Peel and finely slice the onions and garlic. Trim and finely slice the fennel. Coarsely grate all the cheese and leave to one side. Grind the fennel seeds in a pestle and mortar until fine.

Bring the vegetable stock to the boil in a large saucepan. Blanch the shredded cabbage in the stock for 5 minutes, then remove to a bowl with a slotted spoon and set aside. Keep the stock hot in the pan and squeeze in the juice from the lemon half.

Preheat the oven to 180°C/gas 4. Heat a good drizzle of olive oil in a non-stick frying pan. Pick and shred most of the sage leaves (leave a few whole for garnishing) and add to the pan with the garlic. Fry over a medium-low heat for a couple of minutes, until the garlic is golden. Add the sliced fennel, ground fennel seeds, leeks and anchovies and reduce the heat. Sauté for 12–15 minutes, until the veg are soft and sticky but not coloured, and the anchovies have broken down. Add the blanched cabbage to the pan, season well and mix everything together. Remove from the heat.

Cut the bread into 12–15 slices and toast all but 5 of them until golden. Get a wide, deep ovenproof dish (about 25cm across) and start layering up the soup. Start with half the toast, cutting the slices if necessary to create a secure, even layer on the bottom. Top with half of the cabbage and onion mixture, and sprinkle over a third of the grated cheese. Layer with the remaining toast, cabbage and a third more cheese. Ladle over the stock, until the dish is almost full, then finish with a layer of the untoasted bread. Push and submerge the bread into the stock, scatter over the remaining cheese and sage leaves, and drizzle with a little olive oil. Bake in the oven for 20-25 minutes, until the top is golden. Serve immediately.

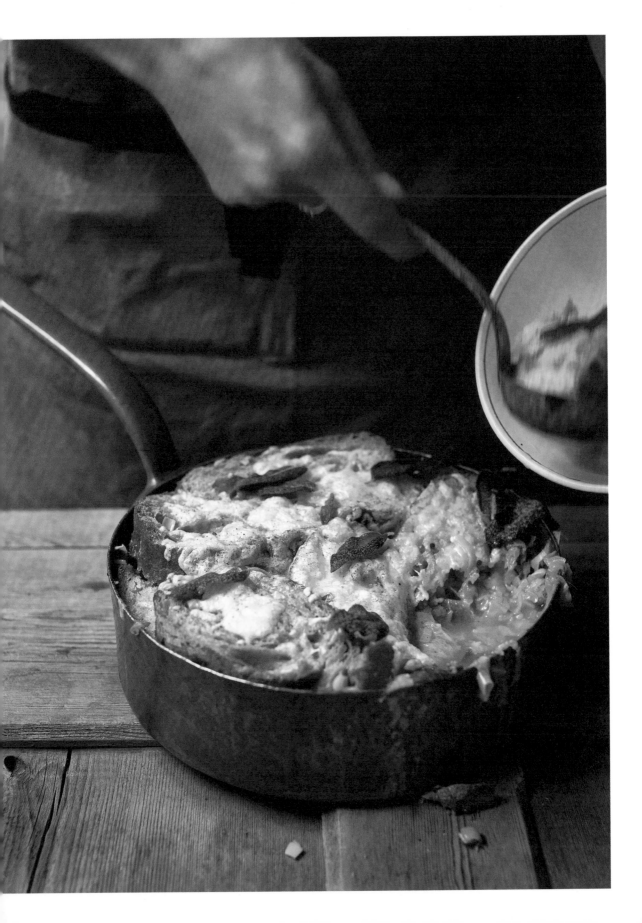

CRAB AND PRAWN WONTON BROTH WITH CHARRED CORN

This soup is so wonderfully simple and pretty that I'm always pleased as punch when I've made it for myself. My tip is when you find wonton wrappers (in Asian supermarkets or online), keep a few packets stored in the freezer, then this becomes a great store cupboard soup. Also, if you don't like crab or prawns, you can use just one or the other. I've even made these with 200g of pork mince before, and it worked just as well.

SERVES 4–6
—

100g crabmeat *(I like to use 50g white meat, 50g brown meat)*

1 tablespoon oyster sauce

1 tablespoon sesame oil

100g cooked prawns

a 2cm piece of ginger

1 garlic clove

24 wonton skins

1.2 litres good-quality fish or chicken stock

2 corn on the cob

2 spring onions

1 tablespoon low-salt soy sauce

sea salt and freshly ground black pepper

1 red chilli

½ a bunch of chives

a punnet of cress

In a mixing bowl mix together the crabmeat, oyster sauce and half the sesame oil. Finely chop the prawns and add to the bowl. Peel the ginger and garlic and finely grate them in, then mix everything together well. Fill a little pot with water and get a tray ready to line up your wontons.

Place a wonton skin on your chopping board, rub the outside edge with a little water and put a teaspoonful of the crab mixture into the middle. Bring the sides up and scrunch together, forming a little bag with a gathered top. (You can fold the wontons however you like, to be honest, as long as they are completely sealed.) Fill all the skins and leave them to one side.

Place a griddle pan on a high heat. Place a large saucepan of water on a high heat and bring to the boil. Put the stock into another saucepan, place on a medium heat, and gently bring to a simmer. Place the corn on the griddle and grill for a few minutes on each side, until charred and cooked through. Stand the cobs upright on your chopping board and carefully cut off the charred kernels. Transfer them to the simmering stock. Trim the spring onions, slice finely, and add to the stock too, along with the soy sauce and the remaining ½ tablespoon of sesame oil. Check the seasoning and tweak to your taste. Halve, deseed and finely slice the chilli and keep to one side. Trim and slice the chives.

When you are ready to serve, pop the wontons into the boiling water and boil until they rise to the surface, which means they are ready. Ladle them into your serving bowls and top with the sweetcorn broth. Finish with the sliced chives, a little sliced chilli and a pinch of cress.

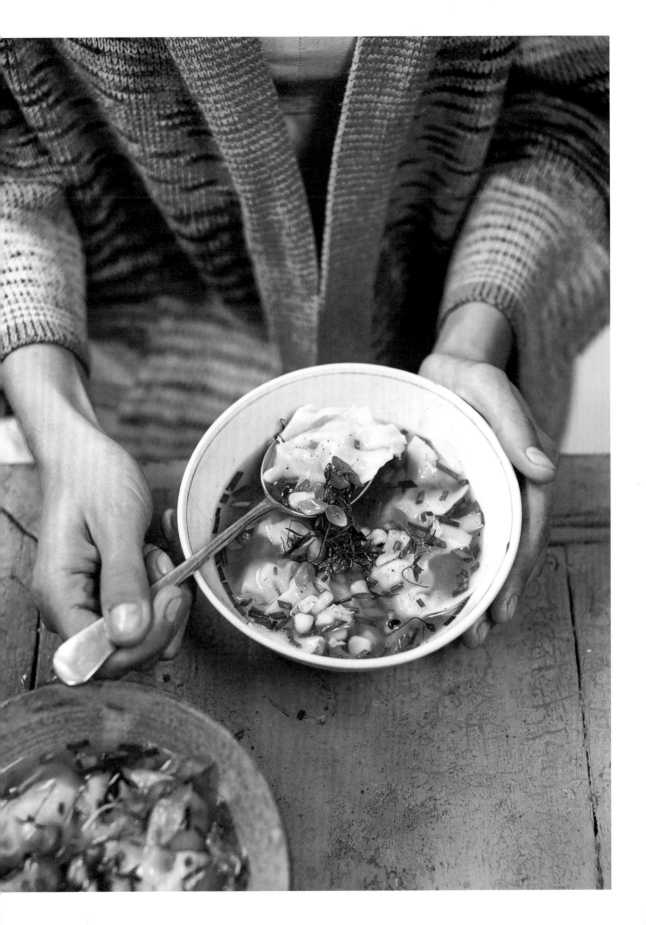

CHICKEN SOUP FOR THE SOUL

This is my recipe for a classic chicken soup, slowly poached and finished with herby dumplings. It's simple and clean and one of the most soothing foods out there. My yiayia and Mum would make this for us, often with rice, if we were poorly, as it's thought to be healing. (The Jewish version, matzo ball soup, is often dubbed Jewish penicillin). Whether it's true or not, there's no denying how comforting this soup is, and the addition of lemon here means it is packed with Vitamin C; great when you're full of cold. So next time you know someone is feeling pants, you know what to cook them.

SERVES 6

—

1 x 1.2kg chicken

2 carrots

2 sticks of celery

2 onions

6 cloves

a few sprigs of thyme

1 fresh bay leaf

½ a bunch of flat-leaf parsley

½ a stick of cinnamon

sea salt and freshly ground black pepper

2 leeks

olive oil

50g chicken fat *(skim it off when you make the broth, or otherwise use 50g butter)*

4 lemons

A few sprigs of mixed soft herbs *(I like a mixture of chives, chervil and dill)*

150g plain flour

1 teaspoon baking powder

1 teaspoon mustard powder

75ml milk

Place the chicken in a large saucepan and pour in enough cool water to cover. Peel and chop the carrots and celery and add to the pan. Peel one of the onions, cut it in half through the root, so it doesn't fall apart, and stud with the cloves. Tie the thyme, bay leaf and half the parsley together with a piece of butcher's string and add to the pan along with the onion halves and cinnamon. Season with pepper and a teaspoon of salt.

Place the pan on a medium heat and gently bring to the boil. Leave the water to gently bubble away for 5 minutes, and skim away any scum that comes to the surface. After 5 minutes, reduce the heat to low and cover with a lid. Gently poach the chicken for around 1 hour, until it is tender and cooked through. If it isn't quite ready, give it an extra 10–15 minutes.

While the chicken is poaching, make the base for your soup. Peel the remaining onion and chop finely. Trim the leeks, removing the outer layers, and finely slice also. Wash them in a colander to remove any dirt. Place a large saucepan on a medium-low heat and add a glug of olive oil. Add the onion and leeks and gently sauté for around 15 minutes, until soft and sticky but not coloured.

Once the chicken is ready, remove it from the broth and leave to one side. Discard the herb bunch, cinnamon and onion halves, and measure the broth. You want 2.4 litres. If there isn't enough, top it up with boiling water. Pour the broth, chopped celery and carrot into the pan with the leeks. Shred all the meat from the chicken, discarding the skin, and add it to the broth. Keep the carcass to make fabulous stock (see page 248). Squeeze in the juice from 3 of the lemons, then taste and tweak the seasoning. Add the juice from the remaining lemon if it needs a little more. Finely »

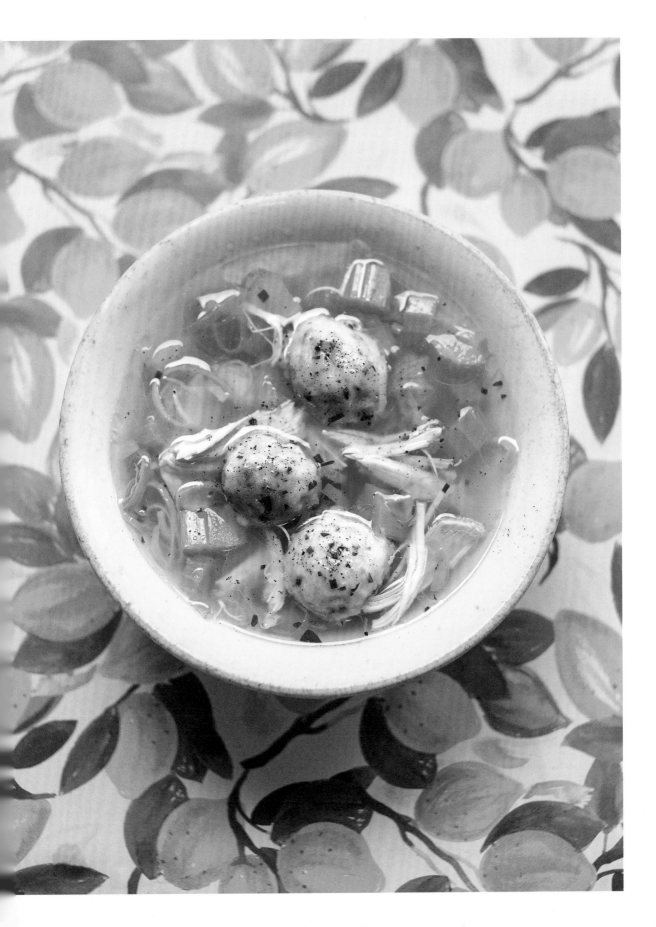

« chop the soft herbs and the rest of the parsley, and mix three-quarters of them in a bowl with the flour, baking powder, mustard powder and a good pinch of salt. Melt the chicken fat or butter in a small pan and pour into the flour mixture along with the milk. Mix just enough to bring together, but be careful to not overwork the mixture. Use a teaspoon to scoop up spoonfuls of dumpling batter and roll into balls – you don't want them too big, as they will puff up. You should get about 24 dumplings from the mixture. Pop these into the broth. Cover for 5 minutes, until the dumplings have cooked through. Ladle the soup into bowls, distributing the dumplings between them, and finish with the remaining chopped herbs.

PORK AND BLACK BEAN SOUP WITH GREEN GODDESS DRESSING

This soup might not be much of a looker, but I promise you it is an absolute corker. Intense, thick and hearty, the green goddess dressing cuts through it beautifully, and makes it a well-rounded meal.

SERVES 6

—

2 green peppers

750g pork shoulder

250g spring greens or chard

2 onions

2 garlic cloves

2 sticks of celery

1 chipotle chilli *(if you can't find chipotle chilli, use a pinch of dried chilli flakes and ½ teaspoon sweet smoked paprika)*

olive oil

2 teaspoons ground cumin

2 teaspoons dried oregano

2 x 400g tins of black beans

750ml good-quality beef or chicken stock

sea salt and freshly ground black pepper

1 avocado

250g natural yoghurt

½ a bunch of coriander

2 limes

50g pumpkin seeds *(or the seed mix on page 82)*

Place the peppers over a direct flame so that they char all over, turning them every couple of minutes (it should take around 10 minutes). When they are ready, pop them into a bowl, cover with clingfilm and leave for 5 minutes.

While the peppers are charring, prepare the soup. Cut the pork into 1-2cm chunks. Trim and shred the greens. Peel and finely chop the onions and garlic. Trim and finely slice the celery. Finely chop the chipotle chilli.

Place a large pot on a medium heat and pour in a good drizzle of olive oil. Add the pork and fry for around 10 minutes, stirring often, until browned all over. Spoon the pork into a bowl and leave to one side. Reduce the heat and add the sliced celery, chopped onion and garlic and sauté gently for 10-15 minutes. Stir in the cumin, oregano and chipotle chilli and stir for 1-2 minutes more.

When the peppers are ready, rub off the blackened skin, remove the stalks and seeds and chop into 1.5cm pieces. Add them to the pot, along with the browned pork, the black beans – juices and all – and the stock. Turn up the heat and bring to the boil. Season and cover with the lid. Reduce the heat to low and simmer for 1 hour. Halfway through, add the shredded greens and stir. Add a splash of water if it looks too thick.

While the soup is cooking, make the dressing. Halve the avocado, discard the stone, and scoop the flesh into a blender. Add the yoghurt, most of the coriander and the juice of both of the limes and blitz. Season to taste and keep to one side. Toast the pumpkin seeds in a frying pan, over a medium-low heat, for around 4-5 minutes, until golden and crisp.

Check the pork after an hour; it should be wonderfully tender. If not, give it a further 10-15 minutes. Ladle the soup into bowls, and finish with a drizzle of the dressing, the seeds and remaining coriander.

PHO FOR ONE

Living in East London near an abundance of Vietnamese restaurants means pho has become a weekly staple in our house (and even prompted a trip to Vietnam). When I am cold/tired/hungry I want pho. It's the childhood comfort food I never had. I've made proper phos, where beef bones are cooked for hours for a rich intense flavour, and there are lots of authentic recipes for that. However, I don't always have the time, and I'm not the person to tell you how to do it. This is my sped-up version, a great 'pho for one' when you are home on your own and want to curl up with something delicious.

SERVES 1

—

1 small onion

a 2cm piece of ginger

650ml good-quality beef stock

1 star anise

1 small cinnamon stick

1 tablespoon fish sauce

100g flat medium-thick rice noodles

a handful of beansprouts

1 spring onion

½ a red chilli *(bird's-eye if you like it hot, regular for a normal heat)*

150g rib-eye, or steak of your choice

groundnut or vegetable oil

salt and freshly ground black pepper

1 teaspoon golden caster sugar

a few sprigs of coriander, mint and Thai basil

½ a lime

sriracha, or other chilli sauce, to serve

Start by charring the onion and ginger. Place them both, unpeeled, over a direct flame on your hob and char them both for around 5-10 minutes, turning occasionally so they're evenly burnt. If you don't have a gas hob, you can do this under the grill. When they are ready, halve them and place in a medium-size saucepan with the stock, star anise, cinnamon stick and fish sauce. Gently bring the broth to the boil, then reduce to a simmer. Leave it ticking away for 30 minutes.

While your broth is simmering, prepare the rest of the ingredients. Cook the noodles according to the packet instructions and refresh in cold water. Place them in your serving bowl. Wash the beansprouts thoroughly, trim and finely slice the spring onion and chilli. Place a small frying pan or griddle on a high heat. Rub the steak with a little oil, salt and pepper, then fry or griddle it for a couple of minutes on each side, until cooked to your liking. (Remember it will continue to cook in the hot broth, so it's best to undercook it a little.) Leave it to rest for a few minutes, then slice it up.

When your broth is ready, stir in the sugar and season to taste, adding a little more fish sauce if needed. Turn the heat up to bring it to the boil again, then strain it into your serving bowl – you should end up with around 400ml of broth. Top with the sliced steak and add the beansprouts, spring onions and sliced chilli. Serve the herbs, lime half and sriracha on the side, and tuck in.

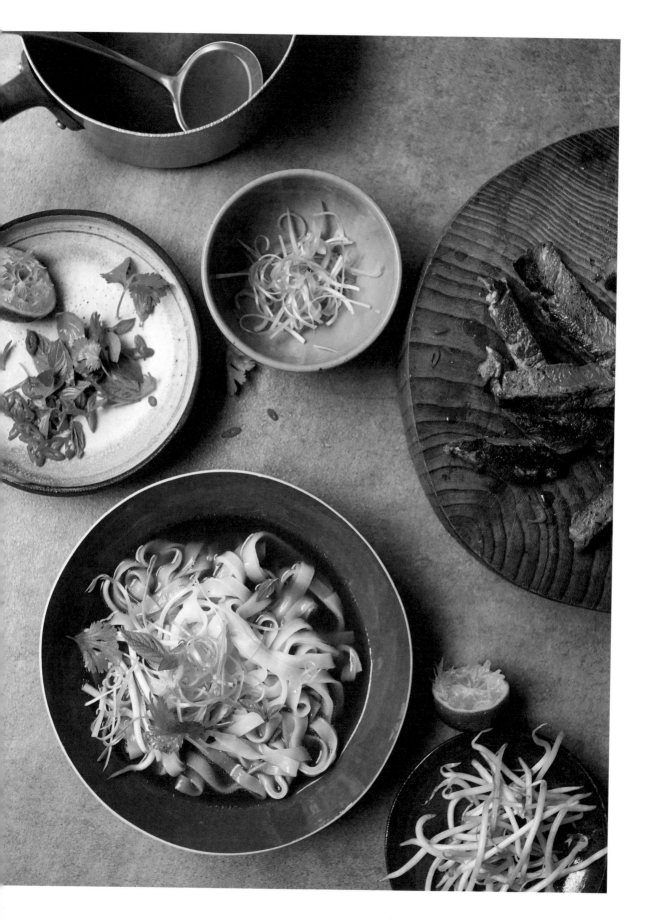

FENNEL AND SAUSAGE MUFFINS

These muffins make a fab accompaniment to most soups, but are also just a great snack on their own – especially if you are entertaining or having a picnic. And if you aren't sure about savoury muffins? I still urge you to give them a go; they're highly addictive, and my once cynical mother is now a total convert.

MAKES 12
—

1 garlic clove

1 teaspoon fennel seeds

200g good-quality sausages, Italian if possible

½ teaspoon dried chilli flakes

150ml olive oil

½ a bunch of spring onions

350g plain flour

1½ tablespoons baking powder

sea salt and freshly ground black pepper

2 large eggs

275ml full-fat milk

135ml buttermilk

200g mature Cheddar

a few sprigs of flat-leaf parsley

Preheat the oven to 180°C/gas 4 and line a muffin tray with cases.

Peel and finely grate or chop the garlic. Grind the fennel seeds in a mortar and pestle. Place a large non-stick frying pan on a medium-high heat. Squeeze the sausage meat out of the skins and place in the pan, along with the garlic, chilli flakes, fennel seeds and a glug of olive oil. Break up with a wooden spoon, and fry until crisp and golden. Spoon the sausage meat on to a plate and leave to one side to cool.

Trim and finely slice the spring onions. Place most of them in a large bowl with the flour, baking powder and a good pinch of sea salt and freshly ground black pepper. In a jug whisk together the eggs, olive oil, milk and buttermilk.

Add most of the cooked and cooled sausage to the flour, and coarsely grate in most of the cheese. Make a well in the middle and pour in the wet ingredients, then pick and finely chop the parsley, add to the bowl and gently fold everything together. Try not to over-mix or you'll end up with tough muffins – a few lumps are OK.

Divide the batter between the cases and top with the remaining spring onions and sausage and grate over the remaining cheese. Bake the muffins for 18–20 minutes, until golden brown and cooked right through. Leave them in the tray for 5 minutes, then transfer to a rack to cool completely.

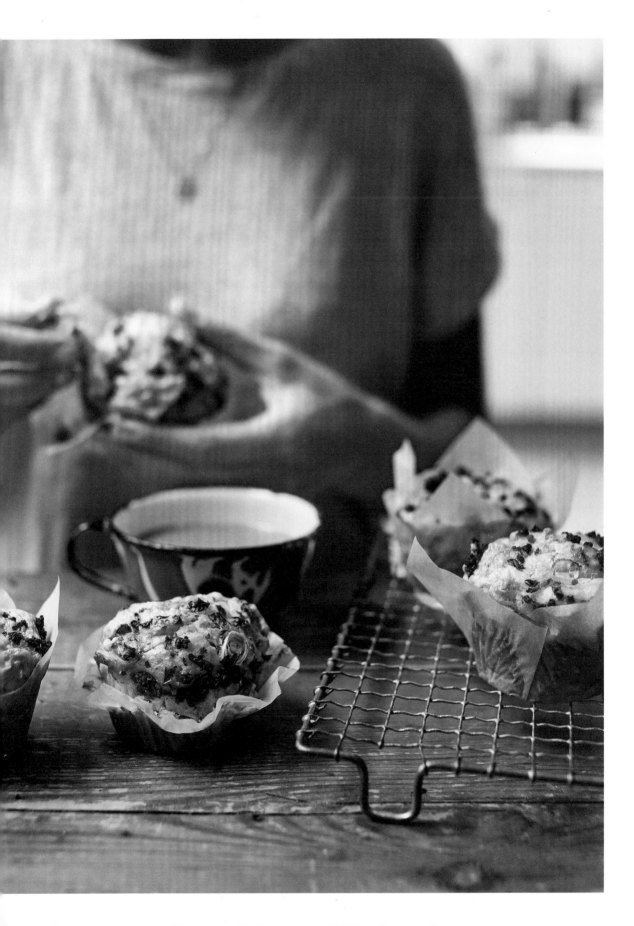

ROASTED SEED SPRINKLE

Dressed and roasted mixed seeds are a great way to pimp up most soups. They last for ages and are a good source of protein.

MAKES ENOUGH FOR 10 SERVINGS
—

1 ½ teaspoons cumin seeds

1 ½ teaspoons coriander seeds

1 ½ teaspoons fennel seeds

sea salt and freshly ground black
  pepper

100g pumpkin seeds

75g sunflower seeds

2 tablespoons sesame seeds

1 tablespoon poppy seeds

1 ½ teaspoons sweet smoked
  paprika

olive oil

Preheat your oven to 180°C/gas 4.

In a mortar and pestle grind the cumin, coriander and fennel seeds to a fine powder with a generous pinch of salt and pepper. Mix with the rest of the seeds and the paprika and drizzle with a good glug of oil. Toss together until coated, then place them well spread out on a baking tray so they are in one layer.

Pop the tray into the oven for 8 minutes, then give the seeds a jiggle and roast for 4–5 minutes more. Leave to cool completely, then store in a sealed container until needed – they'll keep for at least a month. Perfect scattered over soups and even through salads.

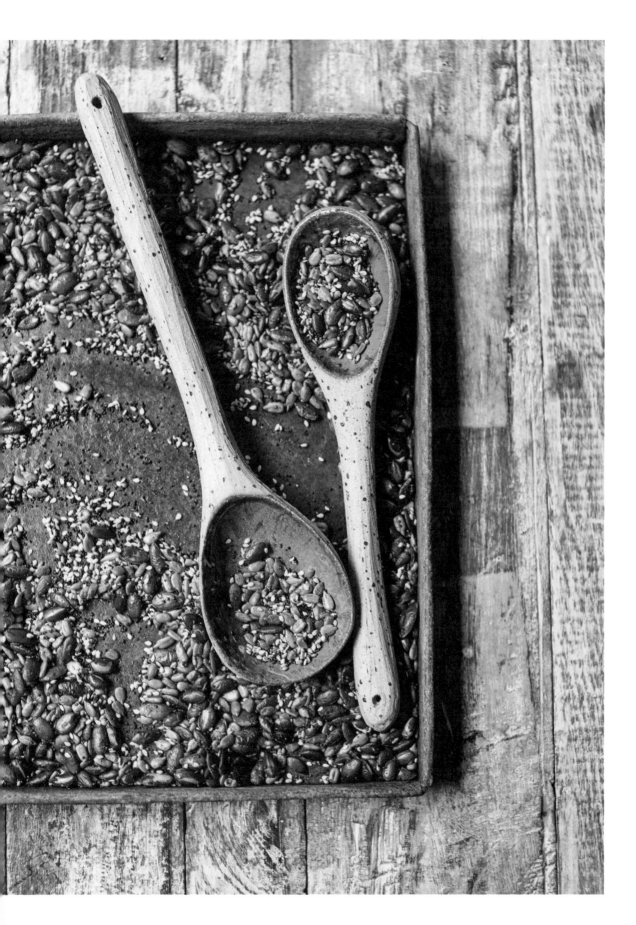

QUICK GRIDDLED MULTIGRAIN FLATBREADS

I love how easy these wholesome, simple flatbreads are and they go with absolutely everything. They're delicious, and filled with fibre – a much better alternative to store-bought bread.

MAKES 8
—

250g wholegrain flour

1 tablespoon oat bran

2 teaspoons baking powder

1 teaspoon sea salt

275g natural yoghurt

Place a griddle pan on a high heat.

In a large mixing bowl mix together the flour, bran, baking powder and salt and whisk together until well combined. Make a well in the middle and pour in the yoghurt. Mix it in with a fork, so it is all combined, then turn the dough out on to a lightly floured surface.

Knead for just a minute, to make sure it is well combined, then roll the dough into a sausage. Cut it in half, then cut each piece into 4. Roll each piece of dough into a ball, then, using a rolling pin, roll it out into a circle, around 1cm thick. Griddle each of the flatbreads for 2–3 minutes on each side, until charred and cooked through. Serve straight away, or wrap in foil and keep warm until they are all cooked.

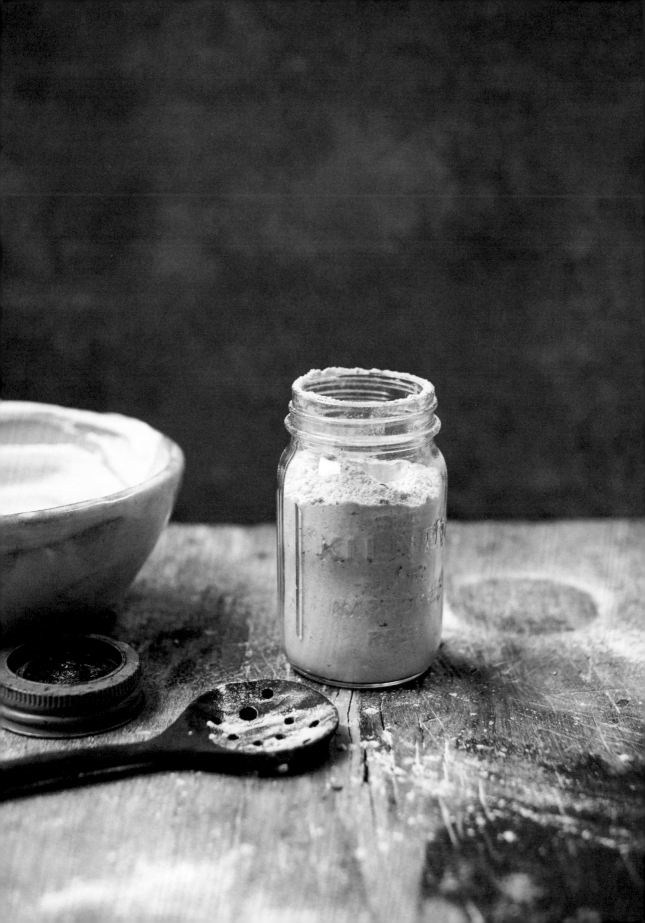

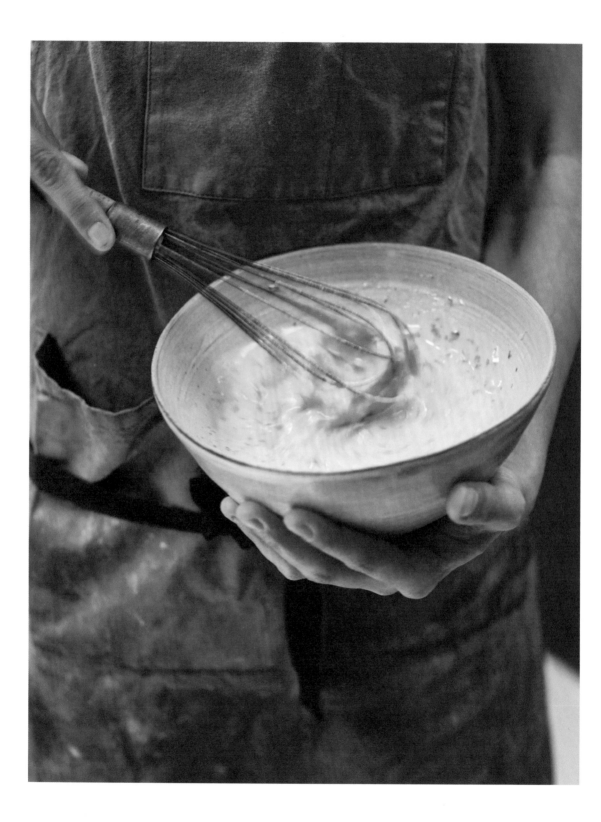

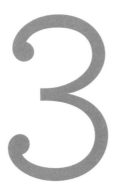

QUICK + LIGHT

—

As with most people, my hunger and
willingness to cook goes up and down; some
days I'm just not that hungry or I don't have
the energy, others my hunger is insatiable
and I want to spend all day slaving over
something incredible. The next two chapters
reflect this. This chapter is made up of recipes
that are easy to prepare, and some that are
light and nutritious. I'm not claiming that
all these dishes will make you look like a
supermodel; however, here is a combination
of quick dishes and recipes that are a little
kinder on the waistline.

LENTIL, FETA AND SPINACH FRITTERS

These Greek-style fritters are a perfect post-work meal; they're easy, quick and full of good stuff (they also make a cracking starter). I'm addicted to their ease and simplicity and will often tweak the flavours with whatever I have to hand (goat's cheese, chunks of halloumi, basil ...).

SERVES 4 (MAKES 12)

—

½ bunch of dill

300g Greek yoghurt

1 small garlic clove

1 lemon

sea salt and freshly ground black pepper

extra virgin olive oil

200g baby leaf spinach

1 x 400g tin of brown lentils

2 large eggs

a few sprigs of flat-leaf parsley

100g feta

75g breadcrumbs

Start by making the yoghurt dip. Pick the dill leaves and finely chop, then place half in a bowl with the Greek yoghurt. Peel and finely grate in the garlic, squeeze in the lemon juice and season well. Pour in a good glug of extra virgin olive oil and mix everything together, then leave to one side.

Pour a drizzle of oil into a large non-stick frying pan and pop on to a medium-low heat. Put the spinach into the pan and cover with a lid. Turn the heat down to low and just keep the spinach there long enough to wilt it down. As soon as it has wilted, pop it into a sieve and leave to one side to cool and drain out the liquid. Wipe the pan and leave it on one side.

Drain the lentils well and put into a food processor. Blitz for 30 seconds or so, until quite creamy, then add one of the eggs and blitz again until smooth. Spoon into a bowl and add the rest of the dill, the remaining egg and a good pinch of salt and pepper. Chop the parsley leaves, crumble the feta and add to the bowl along with the breadcrumbs. Squeeze out the excess liquid from the spinach and chop it up. Add to the bowl and mix everything together well.

Place the frying pan back on a medium heat and add enough olive oil to just cover the base. Using a dessertspoon, scoop up spoonfuls of the lentil mixture and gently place them in the hot oil, flattening them slightly. Fry for 4 minutes on each side, until golden and cooked through.

Serve the fritters hot, with the dill dip and a green salad on the side.

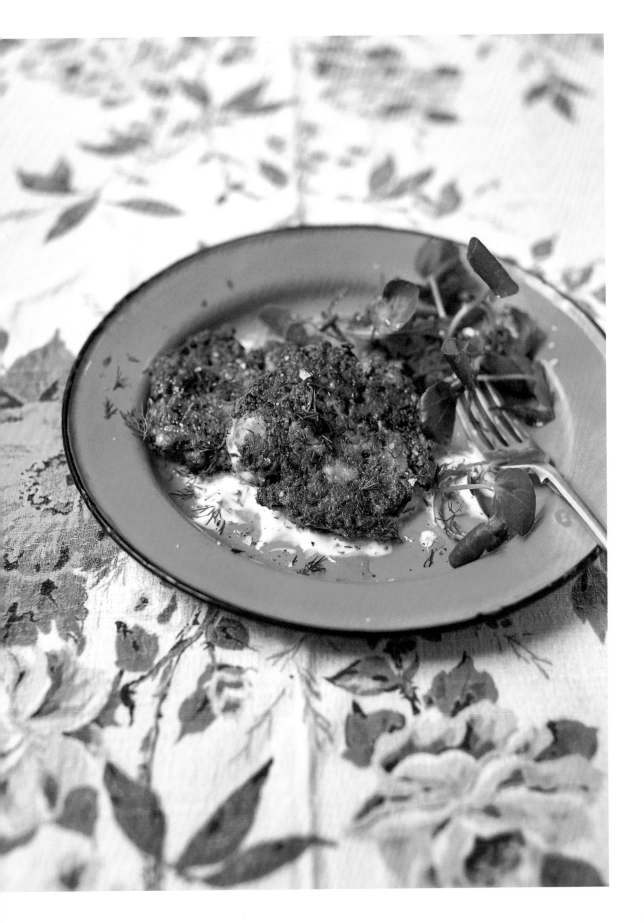

PUDLA

Pudla is an incredible Indian pancake, made with chickpea flour (also known as gram flour). Being gluten and dairy free, it's a great vegan dish, as chickpeas are a good source of protein and will help give you all the nutrients needed for a well-rounded diet. And even if you're not vegan or vegetarian then it's still a delicious and healthy quick meal.

SERVES 4
—

1 red onion

½ a lemon

½ a green chilli

½ a bunch of coriander

½ teaspoon ground coriander

a good pinch of turmeric

250g gram flour

sea salt and freshly ground black pepper

½ teaspoon cumin seeds

3 ripe tomatoes

1 ripe avocado

50g rocket

groundnut oil

good-quality mango chutney

Peel and halve the onion, finely slice half of it, and place in a bowl for the salad. Squeeze the lemon juice over it, mix together and leave to one side. Finely chop the remaining onion half, deseed and finely chop the green chilli and place both in a mixing bowl. Chop the coriander and add most of it to the mixing bowl along with the ground coriander, turmeric, gram flour and a good pinch of salt and pepper.

Place a large non-stick frying pan on a medium-low heat and toast the cumin seeds just for a minute to release their flavour. Add to the bowl with the other ingredients and mix everything together well. Pour in around 300ml of cold water, just enough to make a thin batter that coats the back of your spoon, and whisk together well.

Finish off the salad before you start frying the pancakes. Halve the tomatoes and remove the seeds, then slice into strips. Halve, destone and peel the avocado, then chop into chunks. Add the avocado and tomato to the bowl of sliced onion and toss. You want the avocado to break down and become creamy. Add the remaining chopped coriander and the rocket, and season before tossing together.

Preheat your oven to 150°C/gas 2. Put the same large non-stick pan back on a medium heat and pour in a little drizzle of groundnut oil. I like to spread it around the pan with a piece of kitchen paper, to make sure it is minimal. Pour a ladleful of the batter into the pan, just enough to coat and make a thin pancake, and cook for 2–3 minutes, until golden on one side. Flip over, cook for a further minute, then remove from the pan. Either serve straight away or keep the cooked pancakes warm by wrapping them in foil, as a stack, and putting them in the warm oven.

Serve the pudla with a tablespoon of chutney and filled with the salad.

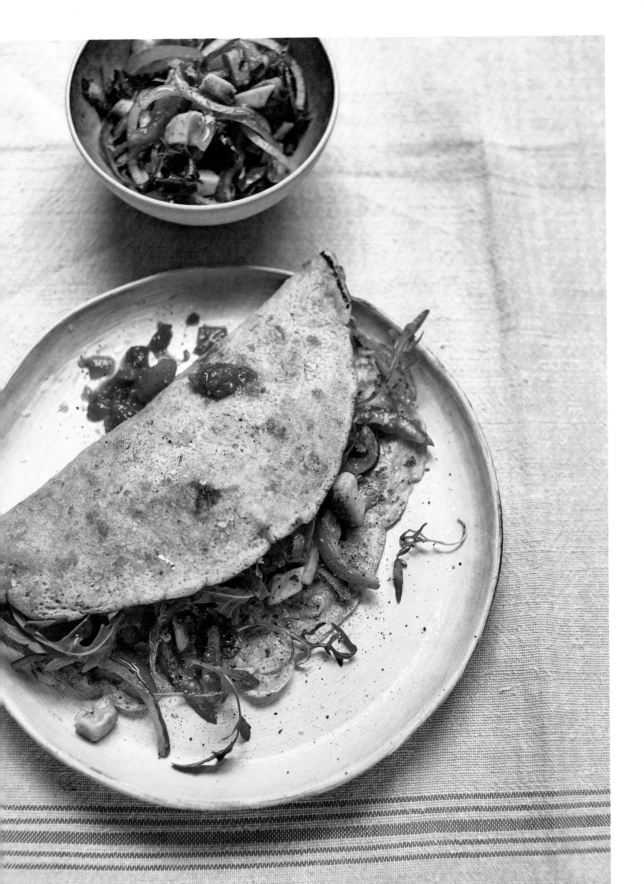

BROCCOLI, KALE AND GORGONZOLA TART WITH GRIDDLED PEARS

This is a wonderfully simple tart that's achievable in not much time at all. The filo makes it lighter than most tarts, with no need for blind baking. However, do leave the tart to rest and firm up a little once it has come out the oven, or the filling will just ooze out as you cut it.

SERVES 6
—

200g tenderstem or purple sprouting broccoli

6 sprigs of thyme

150g natural yoghurt

150g crème fraîche

3 large eggs

sea salt and freshly ground black pepper

1 lemon

75g kale

30g almonds

1 garlic clove

olive oil

250g filo pastry

60g Gorgonzola

3 Conference pears

runny honey

Preheat your oven to 180°C/gas 4. Put a large pan of salted water on to boil. Trim the broccoli stalks and place them in the boiling water for 3 minutes. Drain, leaving the colander or sieve over the steaming pan to steam dry. Then transfer to a piece of kitchen paper to help get rid of any moisture.

Pick the thyme leaves. Place in a large mixing bowl with the yoghurt, crème fraîche, eggs and a good pinch of salt and pepper. Finely grate in the lemon zest and whisk everything together.

Discard any woody stalks from the kale and place the leaves in a food processor. Add the almonds and a good pinch of salt and pepper. Peel and roughly chop the garlic and add also, with a few good glugs of olive oil. Blitz to a fine paste, adding a little more olive oil if the pesto is too thick.

Use a pastry brush to lightly oil a deep loose-bottomed tart tin, around 24cm in diameter. Layer the filo sheets over the base, overlapping them and leaving a slight overhang around the edge, and brushing them with olive oil between the layers as you go. Spoon the kale pesto into the case and spread it out evenly. Pour in the crème fraîche mixture, then line up the blanched broccoli stems. Cut the Gorgonzola into small chunks and dot around the top of the tart. Scrunch any overhanging pastry to create a rim. Place the tin on a baking sheet and bake at the bottom of the oven for 35–40 minutes, until the pastry is golden, the veg poking out is crispy and the filling is just set. Remove from the oven and leave to cool in the tin for at least 10–15 minutes before removing and slicing.

While the tart is cooling, place a griddle pan on a high heat. Cut the pears into quarters and griddle on all sides until nicely charred. Drizzle with honey, and serve a couple of pear wedges with each slice of tart.

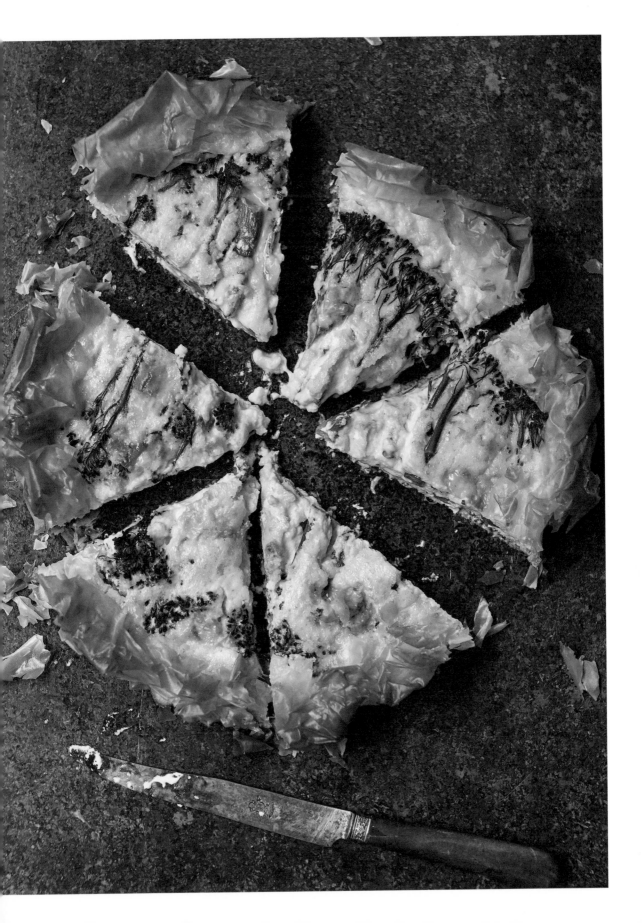

CREAMED GREENS ON TOAST WITH POACHED EGG AND DUKKAH

For me this is pure comfort. I have to stop myself just eating the greens straight up, and actually serve them with something. You can use whatever leaf is available – spinach, kale, chard, cavolo nero, whatever takes your fancy, they're all delicious. I'd avoid baby leaf spinach, though, as it tends to wilt away to nothing.

SERVES 1
—

125g mixed greens *(spinach, kale, chard, cavolo nero)*

a few sprigs of dill

1 shallot

2 garlic cloves

a knob of butter

75ml single cream

sea salt and freshly ground black pepper

nutmeg

25g soft cheese *(I love goat's or blue cheese)*

1 large egg

1 large slice of sourdough bread

extra virgin olive oil

½ a lemon

1 teaspoon homemade dukkah *(see page 258)*

Wash the greens, discard any woody stalks, and chop the leaves – keeping some slightly larger pieces and shredding a few leaves finely.
Pick the dill leaves and chop finely. Peel and finely chop the shallot and 1½ garlic cloves.

Put the butter into a medium non-stick frying pan and pop on to a medium-low heat. Add the shallot and garlic and sauté for 10 minutes, until soft and sticky, but not coloured. Add the chopped greens, stir, then cover with a lid. Reduce the heat and cook the greens for 10 minutes, until they are tender.

While the greens are cooking, fill a small saucepan with salted water and place on a high heat.

When the greens have softened, stir in the cream and dill and season well. Finely grate in a little nutmeg. Crumble in your chosen cheese and remove from the heat. Poach the egg in the boiling water – I like mine cooked for 3 minutes, so the yolk is still a little runny inside. Toast the slice of sourdough.

When everything is ready, place the sourdough on your plate, rub with the cut side of the remaining half garlic clove and drizzle with a little extra virgin olive oil. Top with the creamy garlic greens and squeeze over a little lemon juice. Top with the poached egg and sprinkle over the dukkah. Tuck in.

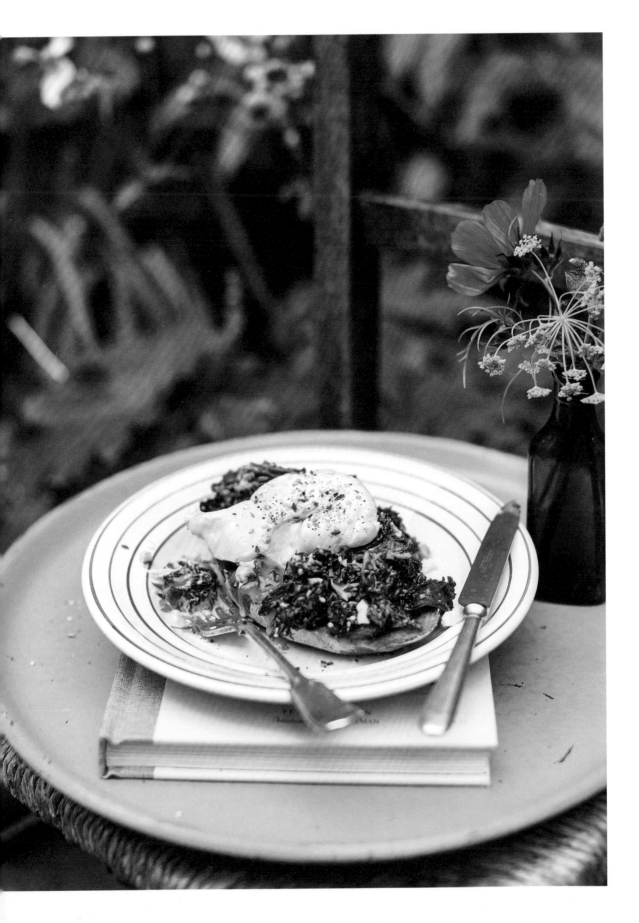

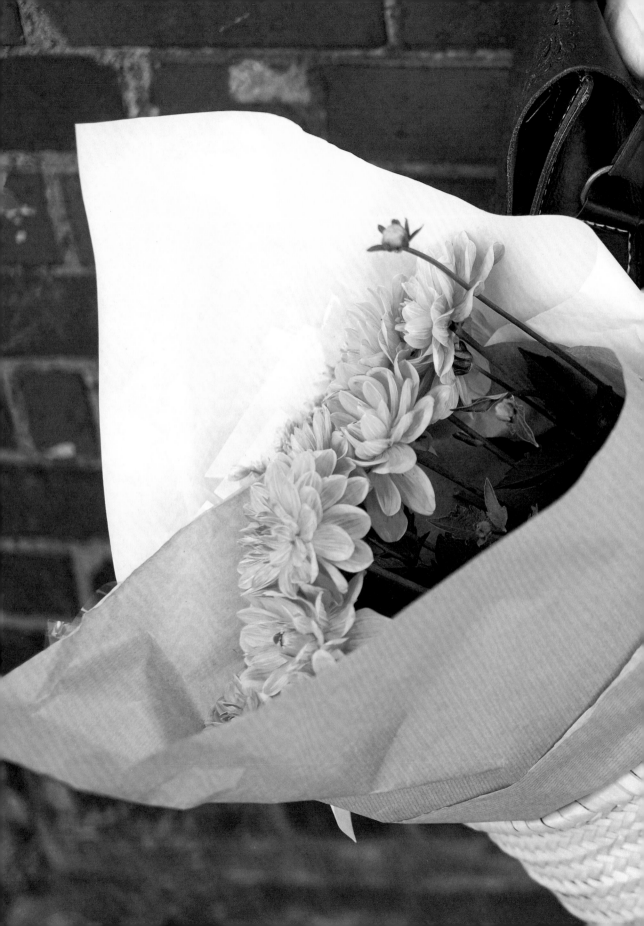

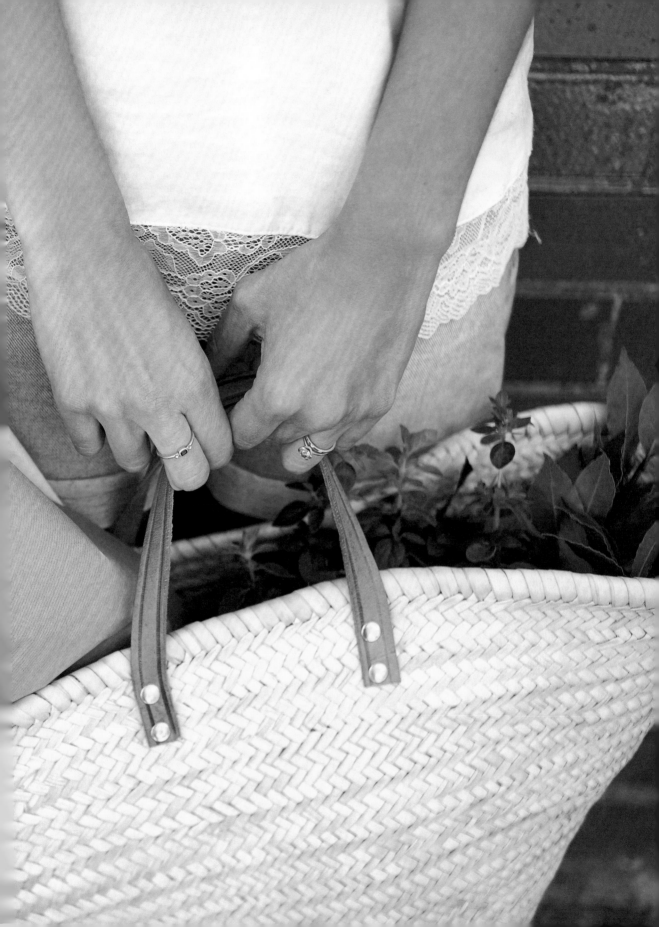

KIMCHI AND PRAWN OKONOMIYAKI

I first tried okonomiyaki at a food market near our home many moons ago, and would drag myself out of bed on Sundays to get my fix. It's essentially a large veg-packed Japanese pancake, which I have simplified to make at home. Kimchi is optional, so don't feel obliged to use it, and try adding different veg (always keeping the cabbage, though). You could even change the protein if you like – shredded pork or beef are great – or leave it out altogether if you're vegetarian (it's seriously good with grated Cheddar). And from start to finish it takes no more than 20 minutes – what a dream.

SERVES 2

—

2 large eggs

150g plain flour

1 teaspoon baking powder

sea salt and freshly ground black pepper

250g Chinese cabbage

60g kimchi

100g small cooked prawns

2 tablespoons sesame seeds

groundnut or rapeseed oil

3 spring onions

1 heaped teaspoon pickled ginger

3 tablespoons okonomiyaki sauce *(or, 1 tablespoon runny honey, 2 teaspoons ketchup, ½ tablespoon Worcestershire sauce, 2 teaspoons low-salt soy sauce)*

3 tablespoons mayonnaise *(ideally from a squeezy bottle)*

2 tablespoons seaweed flakes

a few pinches of bonito flakes

In a large jug or mixing bowl whisk together the eggs, flour, baking powder, a good pinch of salt and pepper and 150ml of water until you have a smooth batter. Trim and finely shred the cabbage and finely slice the kimchi. Mix them into the pancake batter with the prawns.

Place a medium-size non-stick frying pan on a medium heat and add the sesame seeds. Toast them for a couple of minutes until golden, then transfer to a small plate. Place the pan back on the hob and pour in a good glug of oil. Ladle in half the batter and leave it to fry for 6–7 minutes, until golden underneath and just set. Quickly and confidently flip the pancake over and cook for a further 4–5 minutes.

While your pancake is cooking, prepare the garnishes. Finely slice the spring onions and pickled ginger. If you are making your own okonomiyaki sauce, mix the runny honey, ketchup, Worcestershire and soy sauces together. Brush the top of the pancake with half of the okonomiyaki sauce just before serving.

Transfer the glazed pancake to a plate, drizzle with half of the mayonnaise, then sprinkle over the seaweed, ginger, toasted sesame seeds and spring onions, and finish with a pinch of the bonito flakes. Serve immediately, then repeat with the remaining ingredients.

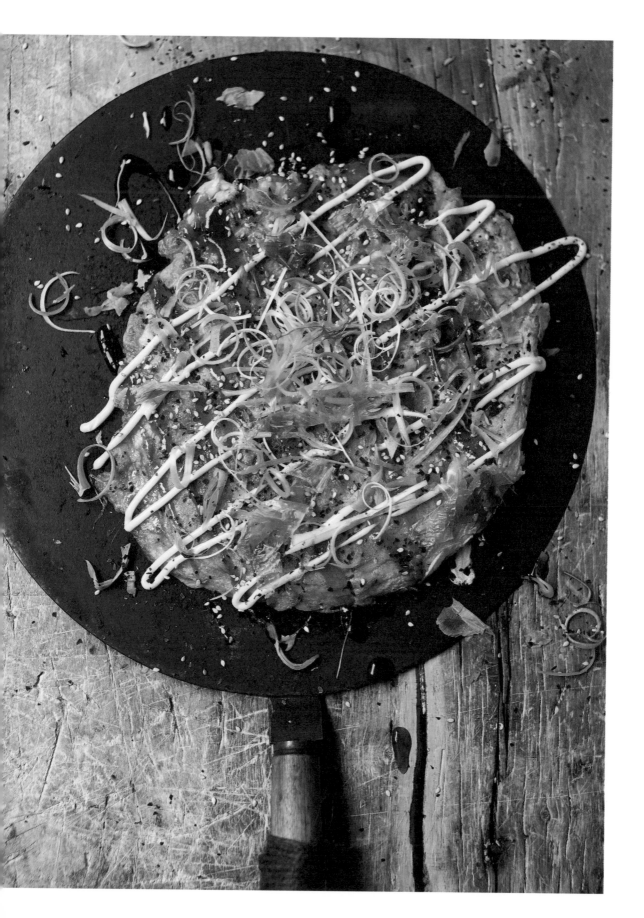

MISO TUNA SARNIE

Sometimes sandwiches are the quickest and easiest form of lunch, but that doesn't mean they have to be boring and/or lardy. Good tuna is a beautiful thing, but drenching it in substandard fatty mayonnaise seems criminal. Try this insanely easy miso-dressed tuna, for a creamy and more flavoursome alternative.

SERVES 1
—

70g good tinned tuna, ideally in olive oil

2 tablespoons natural yoghurt

1 heaped teaspoon sweet white miso

1 teaspoon low-salt soy sauce

sea salt and freshly ground black pepper

½ a ripe avocado

2 slices of your favourite bread

½ a lime

a little salad cress

Drain the tuna of its oil, then spoon it into a small mixing bowl and break it up lightly with a fork. Stir in the yoghurt, miso and soy sauce and mix together well, breaking the tuna even more as you go, until you have a creamy mixture. Season with a little salt and a generous pinch of pepper.

Scoop the avocado straight on to one of your bread slices and lightly mash it into the bread, spreading it as you go. Squeeze over the lime juice and top with the dressed tuna. Garnish with the salad cress, then cover with the second bread slice. Cut in half, and dig in.

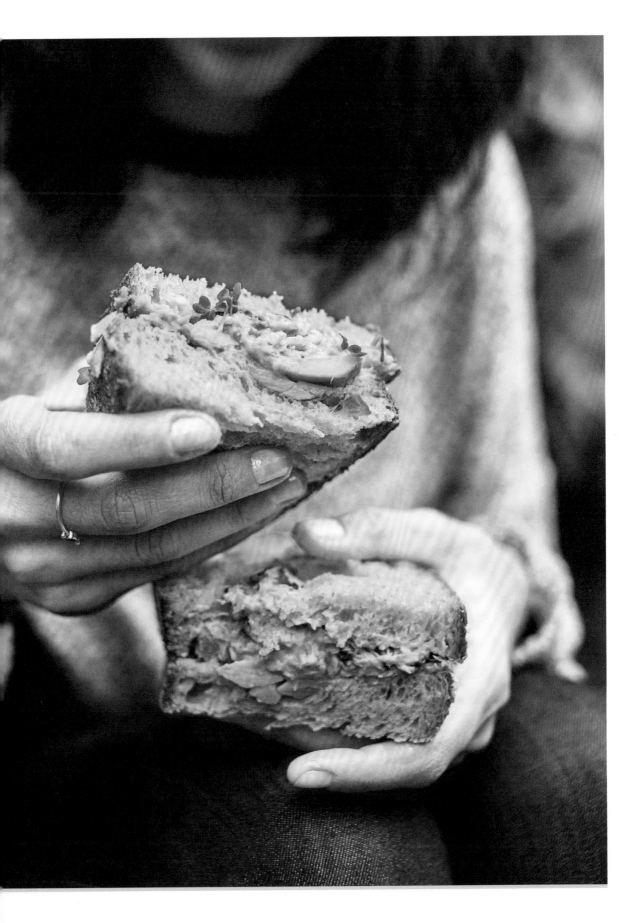

MY FAVOURITE QUICK NOODLE BOWL

This is probably the meal I make most often when I'm home on my own. It takes less than 10 minutes, and for something with so few ingredients it is well tasty. It does rely on you having the chilli oil on page 263 in the cupboard, but I can't big it up enough. It's worth having, to pimp up most dishes.

SERVES 1

—

75g broccoli

75g medium egg noodles

1 spring onion

a few sprigs of soft herbs
(coriander, chives, mint and basil work well)

30g baby leaf spinach

60g leftover cooked meat or tofu
(I particular love shredded ham hock, though any protein will work)

2 tablespoons addictive roasted chilli oil (see page 263)

½ tablespoon low-salt soy sauce

1 lime

½ a ripe avocado

sea salt and freshly ground black pepper

Put a medium-size pan of salted water on to boil on a medium heat. As it comes to the boil, trim the broccoli and cut into even-size florets. Add the broccoli and noodles to the pan and cook for 4 minutes.

While they are cooking, trim and finely slice the spring onion. Pick the herb leaves and finely chop. Roughly chop the spinach, if you like, and shred or cut your chosen protein into bite-size pieces.

As soon as the broccoli and noodles are ready, reserve a splash of the cooking water, then drain in a sieve or colander and return them to the dry pan. Stir in the spinach, chilli oil, soy sauce and sliced spring onion. Squeeze in the lime juice, and use a teaspoon to scoop in nuggets of the avocado. Add the chopped herbs and protein, and stir everything together for a minute, adding a little of the reserved cooking water to loosen – you want the avocado to break down, resulting in a spicy, creamy dressing. Season to taste and tuck in straight away.

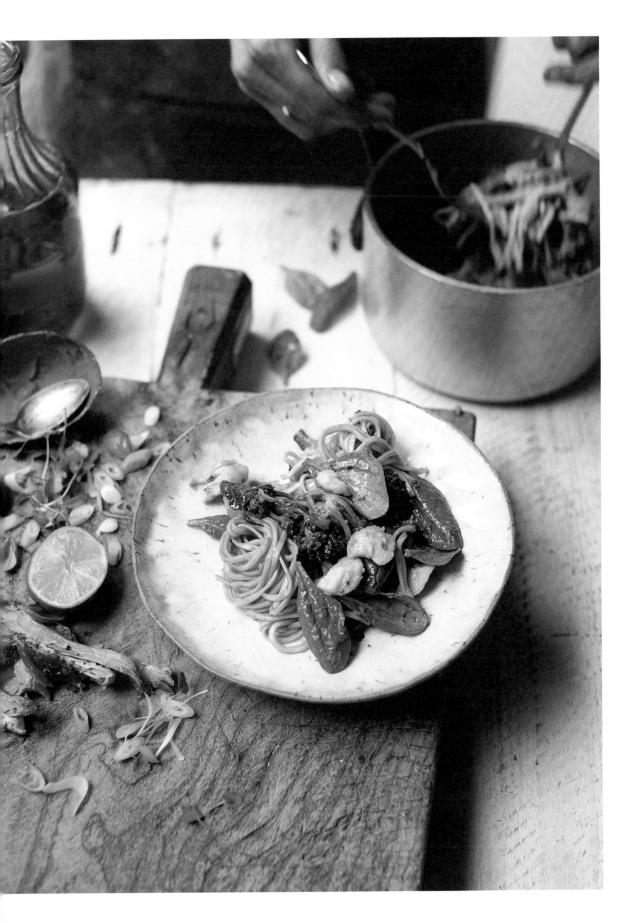

HERBY PUY LENTILS, GREENS AND SMOKED MACKEREL

This recipe started life as an attempt to make myself more intelligent (omega-3s) and boost my iron intake. It turned out to be a wonderfully delicious salad, and so has remained a regular in our week-night repertoire – two birds, one stone.

SERVES 2 (multiply as needed)
—

sea salt and freshly ground black pepper

100g Puy lentils

1 lemon

1 teaspoon English mustard

2 tablespoons extra virgin olive oil

a few sprigs each of mixed soft herbs (*I like a mixture of tarragon, basil, parsley and mint*)

2 spring onions

1 small bulb of fennel

1 ripe avocado

70g baby spinach

150g smoked mackerel (*or if you don't like mackerel or are a vegetarian it's equally delicious with feta*)

1 teaspoon sumac

½ teaspoon black sesame seeds (*you can use regular ones if you can't get black, just toast them first*)

Bring a small pan of salted water to the boil and cook the Puy lentils according to the packet instructions, so they still hold their shape. When they are ready, drain, then leave to steam dry for a few minutes.

While the lentils are cooking you can make the dressing. Squeeze the lemon juice into a large serving bowl, and spoon in the mustard and olive oil. Pick the herbs, discard the stalks and finely chop the leaves. Stir into the dressing along with a good pinch of salt and pepper. Trim and finely slice the spring onions and add to the bowl also.

Trim the fennel and shave as finely as possible, using either a potato peeler or a mandolin. Transfer to a bowl of ice-cold water to crisp up. Halve the avocado, remove the stone and chop into 1cm pieces.

When the Puy lentils are ready and have cooled a little, toss them into the herby dressing, along with the avocado and spinach. Drain the fennel, spin it dry, and add to the bowl also. Break over the mackerel, sprinkle with the sumac and sesame seeds, and serve straight away.

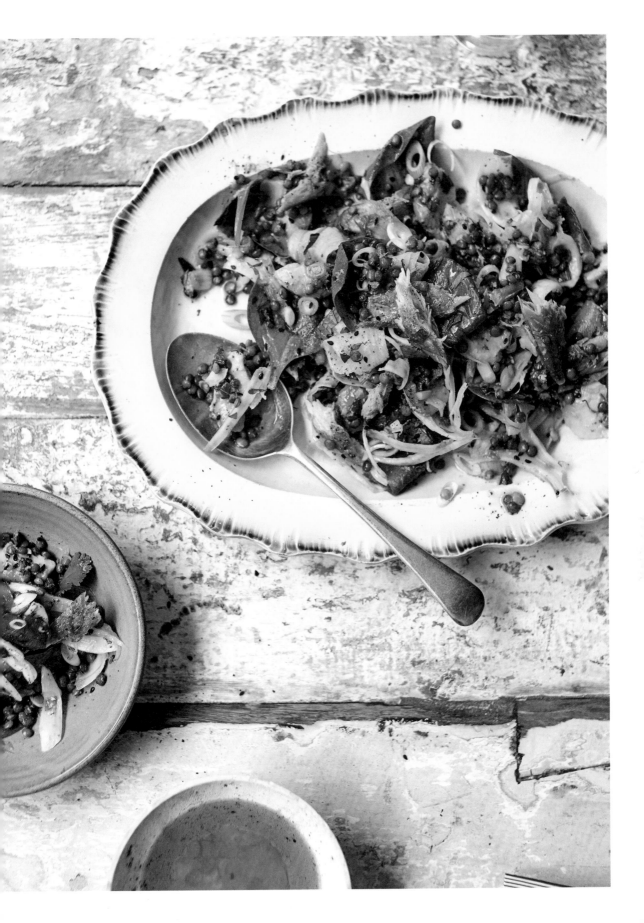

LEMON SOLE WITH PRESERVED LEMON, CORIANDER AND CAPERS

I adore this recipe. It's quick to prepare and quick to cook. If you are rushing you could have this done from start to finish in 15 minutes flat, which for something so flavoursome and nutritious is no mean feat. A perfect lunch or light supper.

SERVES 2
—

125g couscous

250g lemon sole fillets *(you could use plaice too – any fresh flat fish)*

1 preserved lemon

1 tablespoon capers

a bunch of coriander

1 teaspoon ground cumin

1 teaspoon ground coriander

a good pinch of dried chilli flakes

sea salt and freshly ground black pepper

1 small onion

2 garlic cloves

olive oil

150g asparagus

1 small courgette

a handful of baby spinach leaves

1 lemon, plus ½ a lemon to serve

Start by placing a griddle pan on a high heat, so it gets scorching hot. Boil a kettle of water. Pour the couscous into a medium-size bowl, pour over boiling water to come 1cm above the couscous, cover with clingfilm and leave to one side.

Slice the sole into thick goujons (strips). Halve the preserved lemon and remove the seeds, then pop into a mini food processor. Add half the capers, two-thirds of the coriander (stalks and all), the cumin, ground coriander, chilli flakes and some salt and pepper. Peel the onion and garlic, then roughly chop and add to the processor. Drizzle in 2 tablespoons of olive oil and blitz until you have a green paste. Rub half the paste all over the sole goujons and save the other half for another day (in a sealed container in the fridge it should keep for 3–4 days).

Place a large non-stick frying pan on a medium heat and drizzle in a little oil. When it's hot add the sole goujons, skin side down, along with the rest of the capers. Fry for 4–5 minutes, until the skin is golden and crisp, then flip over and cook for a couple more minutes, until cooked through.

While the fish is cooking, prepare the veg. Snap the woody ends off the asparagus and pop the spears on to the hot griddle, charring them for just a minute or so on each side so they still have a bite. Slice the courgette into thin ribbons with a potato peeler and chop the spinach and remaining coriander. Fluff the couscous up with a fork and squeeze in the lemon juice, then pour in a good glug of olive oil and add a pinch of salt and pepper. Chop the asparagus spears when they are ready and stir through the couscous with the rest of the veg. Serve straight away with the pan-fried sole, crispy capers and a wedge of lemon.

***NB** Use the remaining paste to marinate other types of fish; even rubbed on chicken it works a treat.*

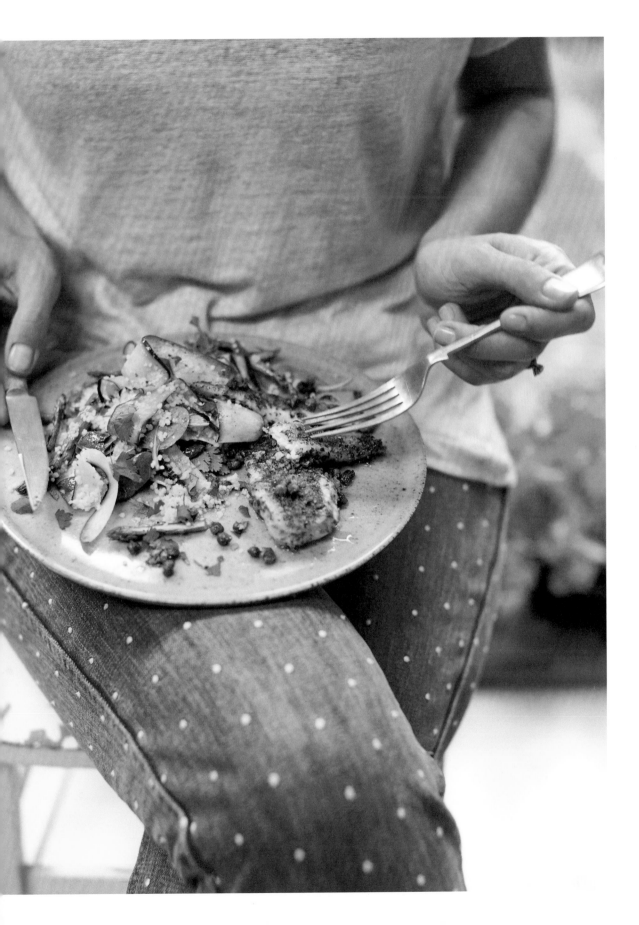

POMEGRANATE CHICKEN SKEWERS WITH WALNUT AND PARSLEY PESTO

I've grown up eating kebabs, and despite the 'dirty late night' connotations, made properly they're a thing of beauty and not dirty at all. Marinated and grilled meat, lemon-dressed shredded veg, pickles, yoghurt and griddled flatbreads – there's a lot of good stuff going on. This recipe celebrates that, while also embracing the delicious kebab elements. It is a cracking crowd-pleaser of a meal.

SERVES 4
—

6 chicken thighs, skinless and boneless

extra virgin olive oil

4 tablespoons pomegranate molasses

2 teaspoons ground cumin

½ teaspoon ground cinnamon

50g walnuts

1 small garlic clove

a large bunch of flat-leaf parsley

½ a lemon

sea salt and freshly ground black pepper

50g kefalotyri or pecorino

1 red onion

250g red cabbage

½ a bunch of mint

1 red chilli

2 tablespoons red wine vinegar

½ a pomegranate *(optional)*

4 flatbreads

Slice the chicken into strips, around 1cm thick and 2–3cm long, and place in a bowl. Toss with a good drizzle of olive oil, the pomegranate molasses, cumin and cinnamon and mix together well. If you have time, leave the chicken to marinate overnight or for a few hours; if not, don't worry, it'll still be delicious. Leave it to one side for 15 minutes. If you are using wooden skewers, soak them in water for at least 10 minutes.

While the chicken is marinating, place the walnuts in a frying pan on a medium-low heat. Toast them lightly, until a little golden, then leave to cool. Peel and chop the garlic. Pop the nuts and garlic into a food processor with half the parsley, the lemon juice and a good pinch of salt and pepper. Finely grate in the kefalotyri or pecorino, add 4 tablespoons of extra virgin olive oil and blitz everything together until you have a thick creamy pesto. If it is a little too thick, add another tablespoon of olive oil.

Peel the onion and finely slice it. Finely slice the red cabbage, either with a mandolin or using a coarse grater. Pick the mint leaves and the rest of the parsley leaves and roughly chop them. Halve, deseed and finely slice the chilli, then place everything in a large mixing bowl and add the red wine vinegar. Season and toss together well, massaging the vinegar into the veg, and leave to one side. If using the pomegranate, remove the seeds and clean them of any pith.

When you are ready, preheat a griddle and heat your oven to 150°C/gas 2. Wrap the flatbreads together in foil and pop into the oven to warm. Divide the chicken between your skewers (either 4 large ones or 8 small), making sure the meat isn't too tightly packed so it has a chance to cook properly. Keep any marinade left in the bowl and use it to coat the chicken as it cooks. Place the threaded skewers on the hot griddle and cook for around »

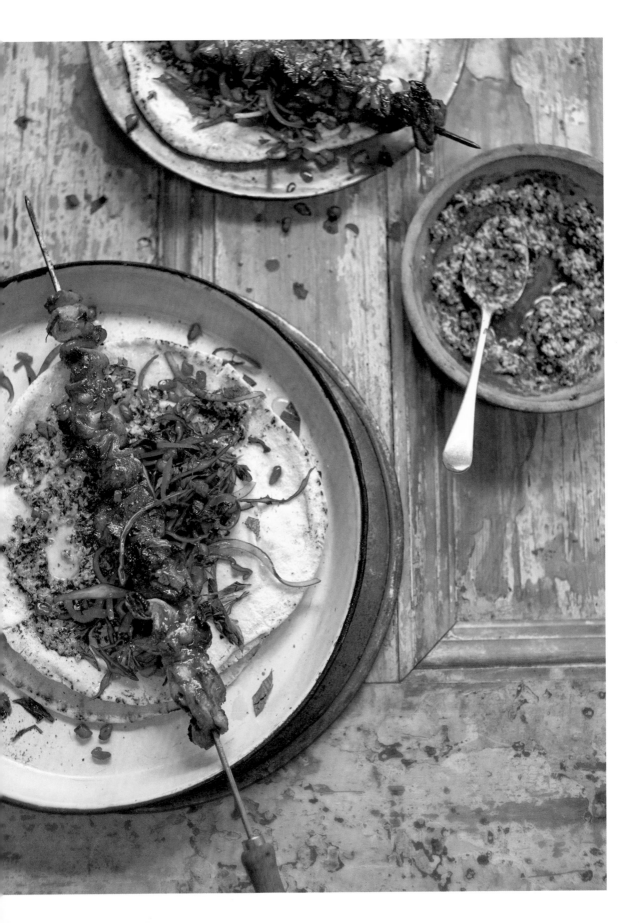

« 2–3 minutes on each side, until gnarly and cooked through but still juicy. Baste the meat with any leftover marinade, and season while cooking.

Serve the hot flatbreads spread with the walnut pesto and topped with the chicken skewers. Serve with the cabbage and onion salad, scatter over the pomegranate seeds if you like, and tuck in.

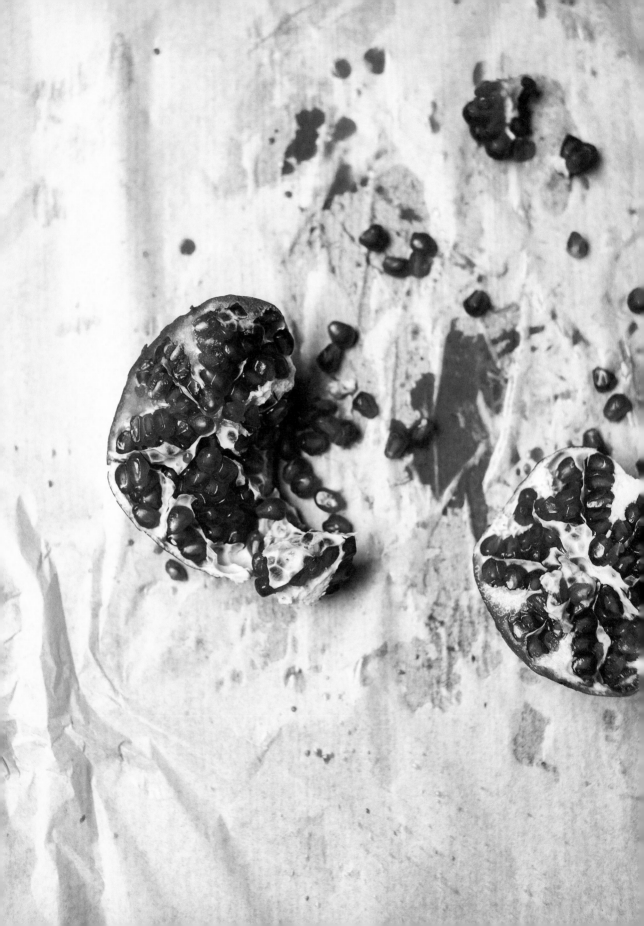

ROASTED STICKY PLUM CHICKEN WITH PICKLED CUCUMBER

This is exactly the kind of meal I want to curl up on the sofa with after a long day. It's warming, sticky and spiced but still light. With this recipe you get that intense sweet plum flavour without having to rely on a jarred sauce.

SERVES 2
—

3 plums

½–1 red chilli

2 garlic cloves

2 chicken legs

1 star anise

1 cinnamon stick

1 teaspoon five-spice

sea salt and freshly ground black
  pepper

groundnut or vegetable oil

a 4cm piece of cucumber

2 spring onions

1 lime

2 tablespoons reduced-salt soy
  sauce

1–2 tablespoons runny honey

150g jasmine rice

1 large or 2 small pak choy

Preheat the oven to 200°/gas 6. Halve, destone and quarter the plums. Halve, deseed and finely slice the chilli. Peel and finely slice the garlic. Place all this in a roasting tray which will snugly hold the chicken, along with the plums, star anise and cinnamon stick. Pop the chicken on top, skin side up. Sprinkle over the five-spice, a good pinch of salt and pepper and a little drizzle of oil, and rub these into the chicken. Spoon a few tablespoons of water into the bottom on the tray to stop the plums burning. Place in the oven for 30 minutes.

Halve the cucumber, scoop out the middle and slice into matchsticks. Trim the spring onions and shred into similar sized slivers. Pop into a small bowl and squeeze over the juice of the lime. Toss together and leave to one side.

Put a medium pan of salted water on to boil. When the chicken has had 30 minutes, remove the tray from the oven and stir the soy sauce into the plum base along with a couple of tablespoons of water to loosen. Drizzle everything with honey and pop back into the oven for 15–20 minutes, until golden and crispy.

Meanwhile, cook the rice in the boiling water. Halve the pak choy if they are small, or quarter a large one. I add mine to the rice pan for the last 4 minutes, or, if you'd rather, you can steam them in a sieve over the top.

When the chicken is ready, remove from the oven and shred the meat off the leg straight into the plum sauce. Taste and tweak the seasoning, adding a little more honey if it needs sweetness or a little more soy for salt.

Drain the rice and divide between two bowls along with the pak choy. Spoon the sticky chicken and plum sauce over the top and finish with the lime-dressed cucumber and spring onions.

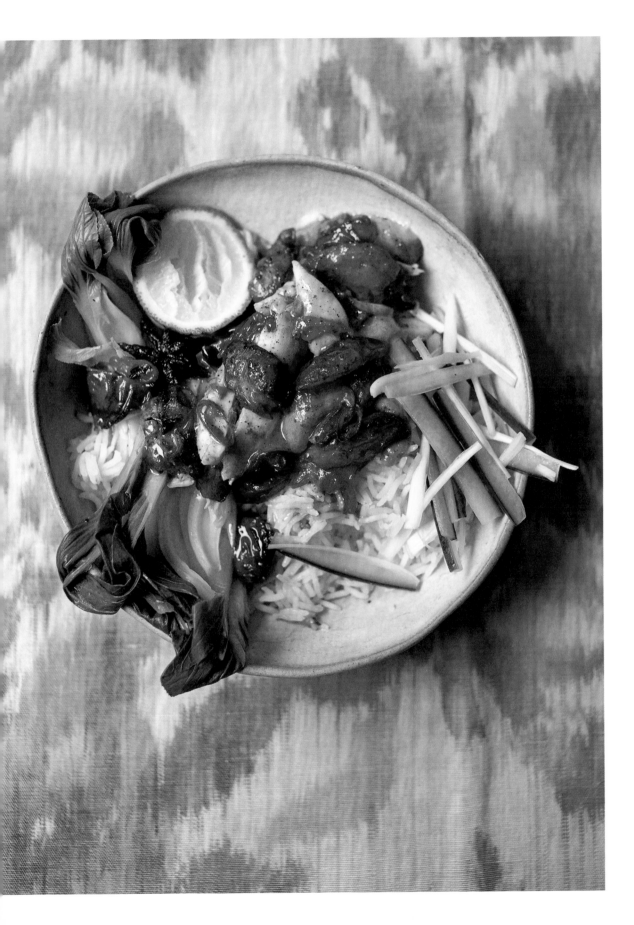

ONE-PAN CREAMY SQUASH PASTA

I grew up eating pasta cooked this way and adore how comforting it is – one pan, no fuss, just rich, creamy and silky. It's not the traditional way, but you have to see it in a different light; it's almost like a risotto, where the pasta creates its own silky sauce from the stock and starch. And as well as being utterly delicious, it isn't too calorific, and you can't beat a bit of one-pan cooking.

SERVES 4

—

½ a butternut squash *(around 600g)*

4 garlic cloves

½ teaspoon dried chilli flakes

1 teaspoon coriander seeds

½ teaspoon ground cinnamon

4 rashers of pancetta *(optional)*

olive oil

1 litre vegetable stock

200g cavolo nero or chard

½ a bunch of basil

320g pasta *(I love shells, or even a mixture of shapes)*

½ a lemon

60g Parmesan

Carefully peel the butternut squash and cut into 1½ cm pieces. Peel and finely slice the garlic. Grind the coriander seeds and chilli flakes to a fine powder in a mortar and pestle. Finely slice the pancetta.

Place a large saucepan on a medium-low heat and add a good glug of olive oil. Fry the pancetta for a few minutes, until golden, then add the sliced garlic for a minute before adding the chopped butternut squash and ground spices. Fry for 4–5 minutes, stirring occasionally, until lightly golden all over. Pour in the stock, turn up the heat and bring to the boil. As soon as the stock starts to bubble, turn the heat down to low and cover with the lid. Cook for 10 minutes.

While the squash is cooking, wash the cavolo nero or chard, discarding the woody stalks. Shred the leaves (if using chard, finely shred the stalk too). Pick the basil leaves and roughly chop them.

Once the squash is ready, stir in the pasta. The stock should just cover the pasta, but if not, add a little more boiling water – you want all the pasta to be submerged. Scatter over the shredded greens and bring back to the boil. Reduce the heat, cover the pan and cook for a couple of minutes less than the full cooking time according to the packet instructions, stirring occasionally.

When the pasta is ready, remove the lid, turn up the heat and continue to cook for a couple of minutes to reduce the stock. Remove the pan from the heat when there is still around 3cm of stock left in the bottom of the pan. Squeeze in the juice from the lemon half and finely grate in the Parmesan. Add the chopped basil and stir everything for a minute till silky and smooth. You'll notice the longer it is off the hob and the more you stir, the creamier and thicker it will get. Season to taste and serve straight away.

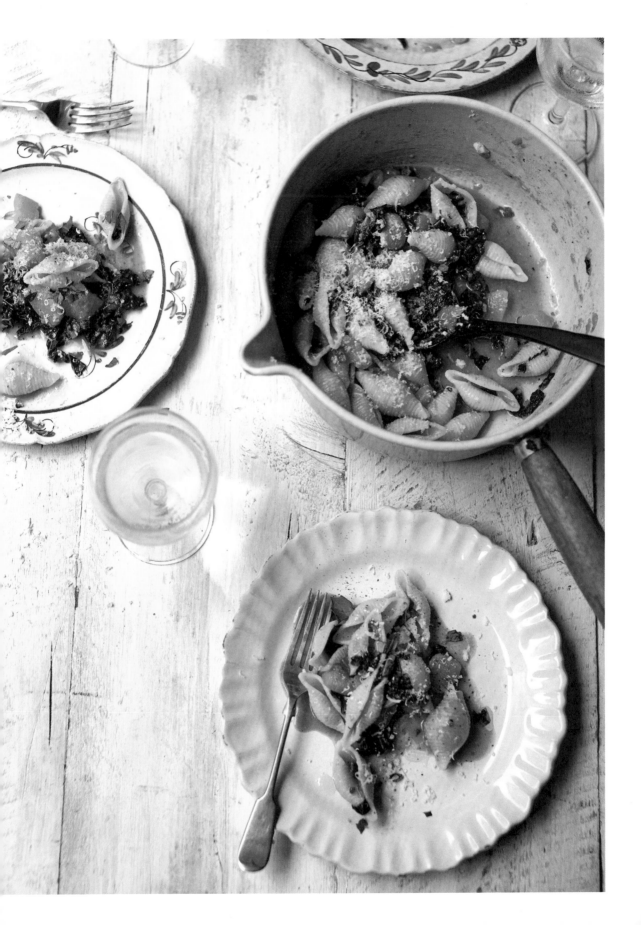

SAUSAGE AND WILD GARLIC LINGUINE

For speed and versatility you can't go wrong with pasta – everyone loves pasta and you can pair it with pretty much anything in the fridge. But this particular recipe is one of my all time favourites: fresh yet hearty and moreish, and it takes less than 15 minutes. Winner.

SERVES 2
—

sea salt and freshly ground black pepper

extra virgin olive oil

3 good-quality sausages (*Italian or something with a bit of a kick works well*)

160g linguine or spaghetti (*I like whole wheat, but you can use whatever you like*)

1 small garlic clove

a few sprigs of basil

60g wild garlic (*if you can't get wild garlic, use baby spinach and a larger clove of garlic; or try sorrel if you can get it, it works wonderfully*)

40g pine nuts

30g salted ricotta or pecorino, plus extra to serve

½ a lemon

Put a large pan of salted water on to boil. Pop a medium-size non-stick frying pan on a medium-low heat and pour in a glug of olive oil. Squeeze the sausage meat out of the skins and roll into small meatballs, about 2cm in size. Pop the meatballs into the frying pan and cook for around 10 minutes, until golden on the outside and cooked through.

Meanwhile cook the pasta according to packet instructions, so it is a little al dente.

While the meatballs and spaghetti are cooking, make the pesto. Peel the garlic and pick the basil leaves. Wash and trim the wild garlic (or spinach) and place in a blender with pine nuts, garlic and basil leaves and 5 tablespoons of extra virgin olive oil. Blitz until you have a smooth pesto, adding a little more olive oil if need be to loosen. Finely grate in the ricotta or pecorino and stir.

When everything is ready, drag the spaghetti from the pot into the frying pan with a pair of tongs, letting any pasta water that's still clinging to it get in there too. Remove the frying pan from the heat, add 2 tablespoons of the pesto and toss everything together well. Add a splash of pasta water as you go, so it becomes super silky smooth. Finely grate over a little lemon zest, and a bit more ricotta or pecorino, and season to taste. Serve immediately.

NB Store any leftover pesto in a bowl or jar, with a layer of extra virgin olive oil on top, in the fridge for up to 5-6 days.

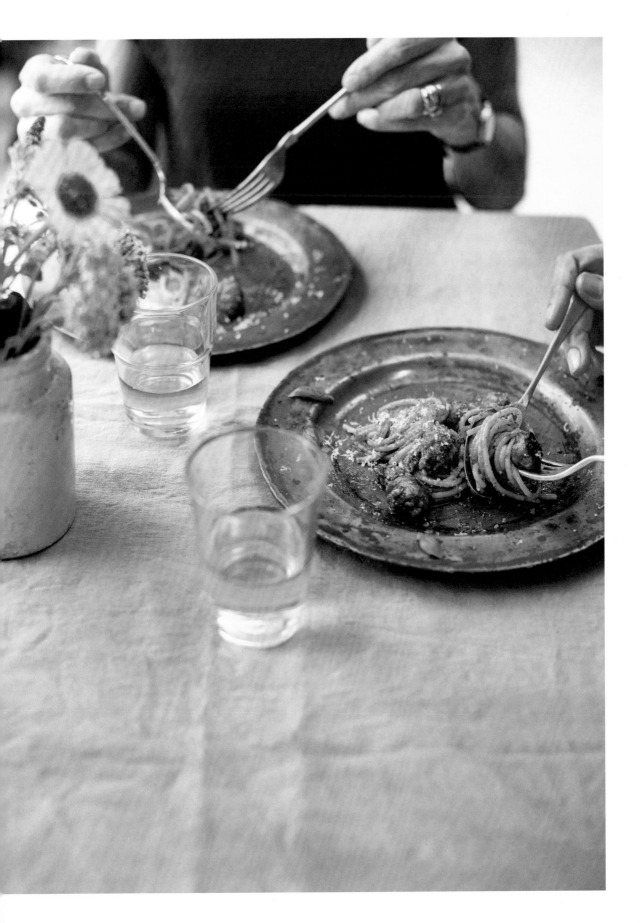

ROASTED CHICKPEA, CAULIFLOWER AND SESAME LAMB

I adore the mixture of textures and flavours in this dish: the crispy lamb, the crunchy celery, the sweet and cool dressing. Perfect with griddled flatbreads and lemon-dressed rocket.

SERVES 2 as a main, 4 as part of a meze

—

1 head of cauliflower, around 750g

1 x 400g tin of chickpeas

1½ teaspoons dried oregano

2 teaspoons cumin seeds

½ teaspoon ground cinnamon

a good pinch of dried red chilli flakes

sea salt and freshly ground black pepper

olive oil

200g lean lamb mince

1 heaped teaspoon sesame seeds

2 medjool dates

1 small garlic clove

2 lemons

1 tablespoon tahini

1 small red onion

2 sticks of celery

a bunch of flat-leaf parsley

Preheat the oven to 200°C/gas 6.

Trim the base of the cauliflower and cut it into even-size florets, cutting the stalks into slices. Put them into a large roasting tray. Drain and rinse the chickpeas and add to the tray also. Mix the oregano, cumin, cinnamon and chilli together with a good pinch of salt and pepper, and evenly sprinkle over the tray. Drizzle everything with a good glug of olive oil and toss together until well dressed. Place the tray in the oven and roast for 30 minutes, until both the cauliflower and the chickpeas are golden and crispy.

While the tray is in the oven, fry the lamb. Place a large non-stick frying pan on a medium heat and drizzle in just a little olive oil. Crumble in the lamb mince and fry for around 12–15 minutes, stirring and breaking it up often, until fine and crispy. Add the sesame seeds for the last 5 minutes.

Remove the stones from the dates. Peel the garlic and finely grate into a blender, then squeeze in the juice of 1 of the lemons. Add the tahini, 2 tablespoons of olive oil, a good splash of water and the dates. Blitz until smooth, adding more water if too thick, and season to taste.

Peel the red onion and finely slice along with the celery. Pick and chop the parsley leaves and spoon everything into a bowl. Squeeze over the juice of the remaining lemon and toss everything together.

When everything is ready, spoon the dressing over a large platter. Top with the crispy cauliflower, chickpeas and lamb. Sprinkle over the parsley, celery and onion mix, drizzling over the lemon juice left in the bowl, and serve.

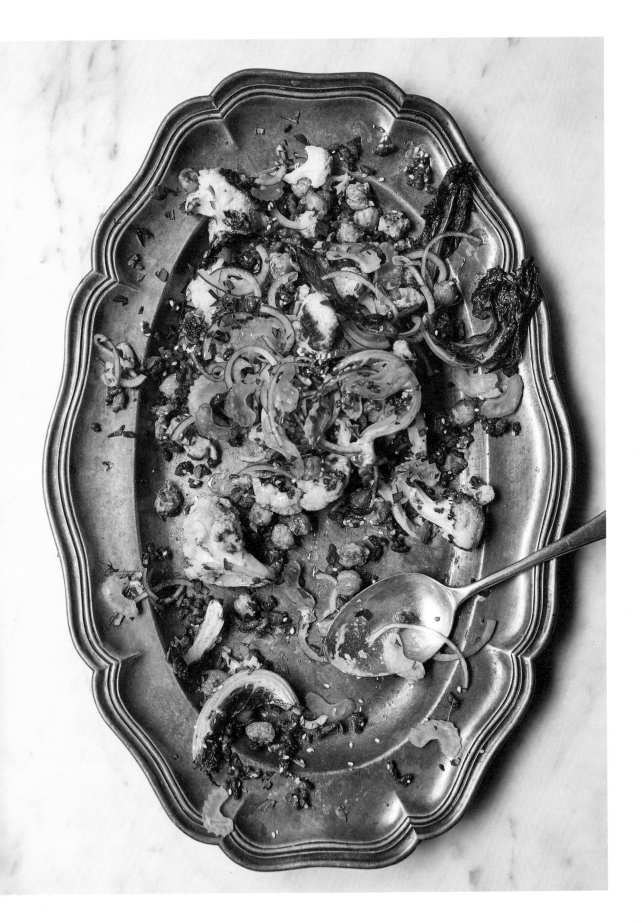

STICKY SPICED MEATBALLS, NOODLES AND PICKLED WATERMELON

This has become a massive hit in our house, and despite the long-ish ingredients list it isn't difficult to prepare. Do go the whole hog and make the pickled watermelon – it cuts through the punchy meatballs perfectly and is such a brilliantly simple side.

SERVES 4
—

50g peanuts

800g watermelon

3 limes

3 spring onions

1 tablespoon rice vinegar

4cm piece of ginger

1 bunch of coriander

½ a bunch of mint

2 shallots

2 garlic cloves

1 stick of lemongrass

1 red chilli

400g lean beef mince *(you could use pork if you prefer)*

2 tablespoons fish sauce

sea salt and freshly ground black pepper

1 large egg

1 heaped tablespoon cornflour

groundnut oil

2 tablespoons honey

250g fine or medium egg noodles

2 tablespoons low-salt soy sauce

Preheat the oven to 180°C/gas 4. Scatter the peanuts into a small roasting tray and pop into the oven for 5–6 minutes, until lightly golden. Once cool, roughly chop and leave to one side.

Remove the watermelon rind, cut the flesh into 2cm pieces, removing any obvious black seeds as you go, and place in a bowl with the juice of 2 of the limes. Trim and finely slice the spring onions and toss into the watermelon with the rice vinegar. Peel the ginger and finely grate half over the watermelon, then toss together and pop into the fridge to chill (you can do this in advance if you like – tastes even better after a few hours). Pick the coriander and mint leaves and leave to one side.

Peel and finely chop the shallots, garlic, the remaining ginger, the lemongrass (discarding the outer layer), the chilli and most of the coriander leaves, either by hand or by blitzing in a food processor. Mix or pulse in the beef mince, fish sauce and a good pinch of pepper until you have a smooth, even mince. Add the egg and cornflour and mix it all together well. Use a dessertspoon to scoop up the mince and roll it into balls, around 3–4cm in diameter. You should end up with around 32.

Place a large saucepan of salted water on a high heat. Pour a couple of glugs of groundnut oil into a large non-stick frying pan and place it on a medium-low heat. Fry the meatballs for around 12–15 minutes, until golden all over and cooked through, then drizzle with honey and cook for a minute or two longer, until the meatballs are sticky on the outside.

When the meatballs are almost ready, cook the noodles in the boiling water, according to the packet instructions. When they're ready, drain and toss them with the meatballs in the frying pan, along with the soy sauce. Serve scattered with the remaining picked herbs. Stir the chopped peanuts into the pickled watermelon and serve on the side.

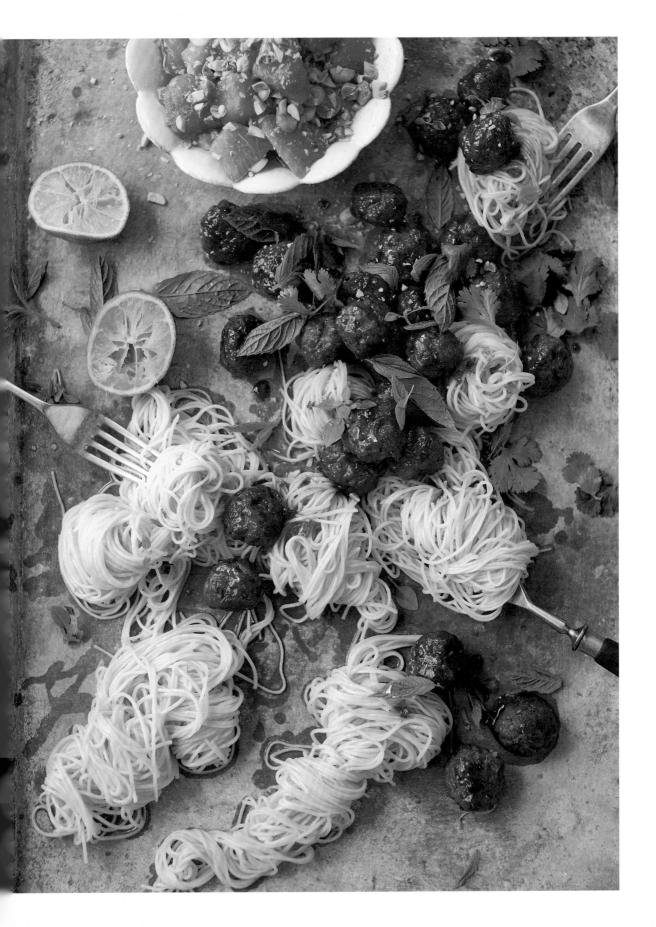

BRESAOLA WITH SHAVED CELERIAC AND HAZELNUTS

The creamy, punchy dressing used here tastes too good to be considered anything other than indulgent, but I assure you it's not. Using yoghurt as the base makes the dressing a little lighter, without scrimping on flavour. Such a delicious light meal.

SERVES 4

—

40g hazelnuts

½ a bunch of parsley

1 medium celeriac, around 700g

1 bunch of radishes

2 garlic cloves

sea salt and freshly ground black pepper

3 anchovies

40g Parmesan

1 lemon

3 tablespoons natural yoghurt

2 garlic cloves

extra virgin olive oil

a loaf of ciabatta

16 slices of bresaola, around 90g

Preheat your oven to 180°C/gas 4. Scatter the hazelnuts into a small roasting tray and pop into the oven for just 8 minutes, until golden all over. Leave to one side to cool completely, then roughly chop them. Pick the parsley leaves and finely chop them, then leave them to one side also.

Peel the celeriac and slice as finely as possible, using either a mandolin or the slicing attachment on a food processor. Put them into a bowl of ice-cold water. Trim the radishes and roughly chop them, then pop them into a mortar and pestle and bash them slightly to break them down a little. Scoop them on to a large platter.

Peel one of the garlic cloves, put it into the mortar with a pinch of salt and crush until creamy. Add the anchovies and muddle them in, until you have a paste. Finely grate in the Parmesan, squeeze in the juice of the lemon, add the yoghurt and a glug of extra virgin olive oil and mix it all together with the pestle. Season to taste.

Place a griddle pan on a high heat. Cut the ciabatta into 1½ cm slices and griddle on both sides until charred. Cut the remaining garlic clove in half and rub the cut side over the charred bread, then drizzle with a little extra virgin olive oil.

When you are ready to dress the salad, drain the celeriac and spin until dry, then add to the platter of radishes. Spoon over the yoghurt dressing, add the chopped parsley and toss everything together with your hands – you want to really work the dressing into the veg. Lay the bresaola around the edge of the platter and sprinkle everything with the chopped nuts. Serve with a stack of the freshly grilled ciabatta.

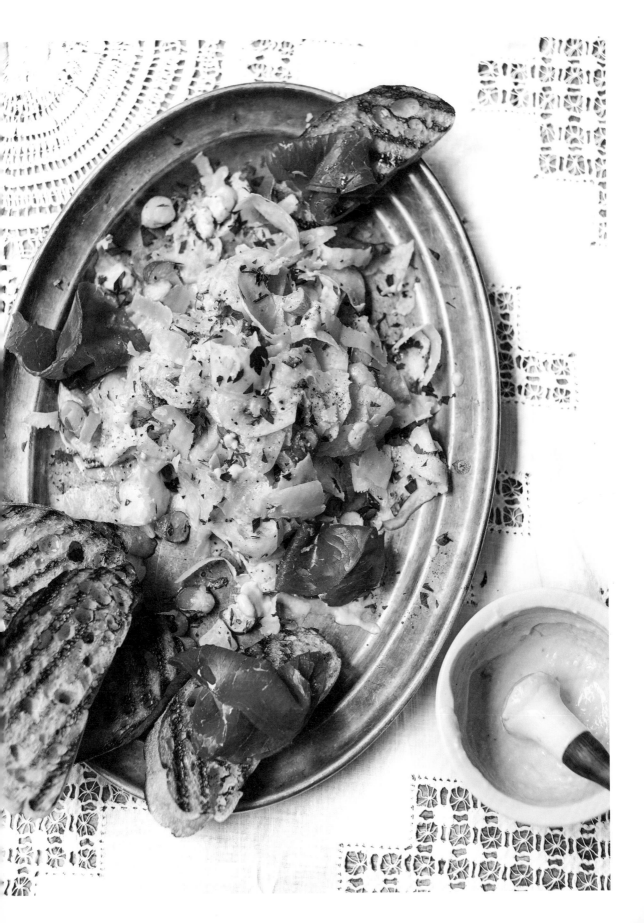

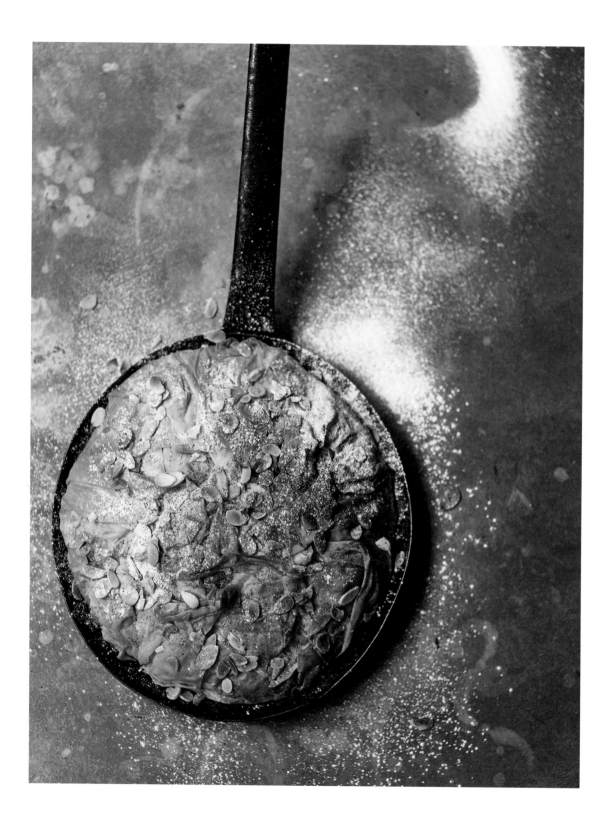

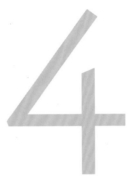

LOW, SLOW + HEARTY

—

This chapter is for the days when you are curled up at home, don't want to go out, and have time to really dedicate to your kitchen. Or just for when you want to indulge in something that is the edible equivalent of a hug from the inside. A chapter of hearty meals and meals that take a little longer; labours of love that require attention and patience and will repay you with incredible flavour.

BLACK DAL

A hugely popular choice with Indian food fans everywhere, this is my favourite way to cook black dal. Slow and low, this is all the better for the hours you give it. An incredibly rich and creamy dish. You can easily halve this recipe, but for the time and effort it is worth making a large batch and freezing any extra for a rainy day.

SERVES 8–10
—

500g urad dal (black lentils)

2 large onions

12 garlic cloves

a 6cm piece of ginger

50g butter

1 teaspoon ground cumin

1 heaped teaspoon mild chilli powder

1 heaped tablespoon tomato purée

1 x 400g tin of good-quality plum tomatoes

sea salt and freshly ground black pepper

500ml full fat milk

double cream or Greek yoghurt, to serve *(optional)*

Thoroughly rinse the dal and then soak it in plenty of water the night before you want to cook it. The next day, drain off the soaking water and place the soaked dal in a large saucepan. Cover with plenty of fresh water, bring to the boil, then simmer for 40 minutes (scooping off any scum that comes to the surface) until the dal is soft.

Peel and finely chop the onions, garlic and ginger. Melt the butter in a large non-stick saucepan over a medium-low heat. Add the chopped veg and soften for 10–15 minutes, so they are soft but not coloured. Add the cumin and chilli powder to the pan and cook for 2 minutes, then add the tomato purée. Cook for a few more minutes, then add the tinned tomatoes, gently crushing them to break them down, and bring to a simmer. Cook for 3–4 minutes, then season generously.

When the dal is cooked, drain and add to the pan of veg. Pour in the milk and top with enough water to just cover the dal. Bring the mixture to the boil, giving everything a good stir, then reduce the heat to low, so it is gently simmering away. This is where you need time. You could cook this for 3–4 hours and it would be OK. But don't settle for that – you want crazy delicious dal and for that you need to cook it for at least 6 hours. Seven if you can. Eight would be amazing. Or keep going – it just gets better...

Leave the dal ticking away uncovered, giving it a stir every now and then. If it looks like it's getting too dry, top it up with a bit more milk, or a bit more water, alternating the two. After a few hours you'll notice it starting to darken, which is great – let it get darker and thicker (try not to drown it in too much liquid) and keep stirring.

Check the seasoning – it is a vast amount of dal, so don't be surprised if it needs more salt and pepper. Serve with a swirl of cream or Greek yoghurt, and steaming basmati rice and chapati on the side.

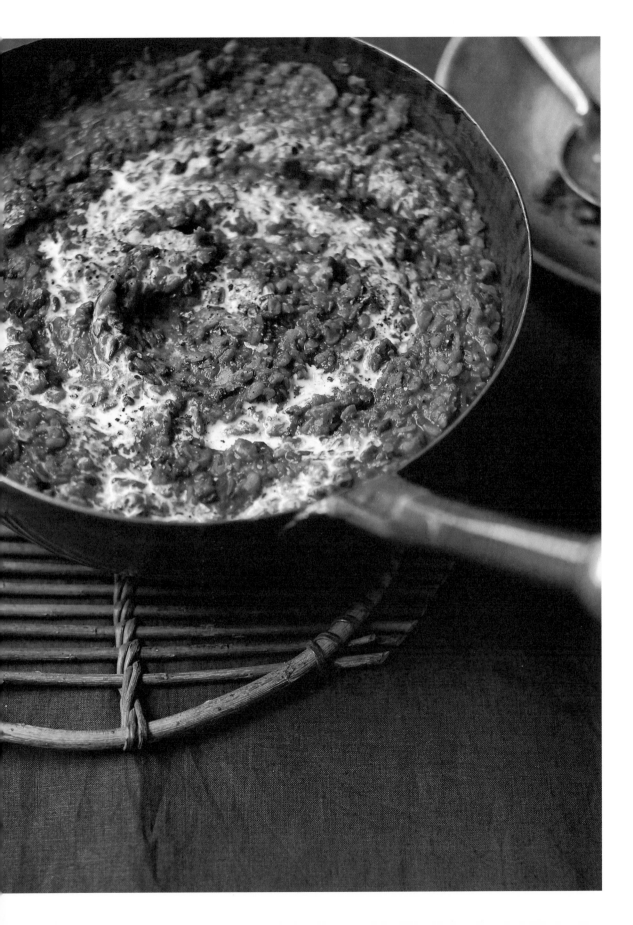

SPINACH AND BASIL GNUDI

The first time I had gnudi was at the Spotted Pig in New York, where the incredible April Bloomfield has made them since day one – and can't take them off. And I can see why. Loosely translated to mean 'naked' in Italian, gnudi are little ricotta dumplings, a bit like the filling in ravioli, just minus the pasta. They're delicate, pillowy and light, and make a fantastic starter or light meal. Be warned that although making gnudi couldn't be easier or quicker, they do need a long time to rest in the fridge.

SERVES 6
—

350g ricotta

a bunch of basil

75g baby leaf spinach

125g Parmesan

nutmeg

sea salt and freshly ground black
  pepper

500g semolina flour

50g pine nuts

25g butter

1 lemon

Drain the ricotta in a sieve, gently pressing out any excess water. Pick the basil leaves, put most of them into a food processor with the spinach, and blitz till roughly chopped. Add 100g of the ricotta and pulse until you have a purée, then spoon it into a large mixing bowl. Add the rest of the ricotta, finely grate in 100g of Parmesan and a good few gratings of nutmeg. Season generously, and beat thoroughly until light in texture. If the mixture feels soft, place the bowl in the fridge for 20 minutes to firm up.

Take a large roasting tray and pour in half the semolina flour. Using a teaspoon, scoop up pieces of the ricotta mixture and lightly roll them into balls, about 2½cm in size; the mixture will be very damp, so don't worry if they are not perfect – the more rustic the better. Pop them into the tray and continue until all the mixture has been used up. Cover the gnudi with the remaining semolina flour, so they are all completely covered and not touching each other. Put the uncovered tray into the fridge for 36–48 hours; the longer you leave them the more robust they will be – it will give the gnudi enough time to form a good semolina crust.

When you are ready to cook your gnudi, bring a large pan of salted water to the boil. Put a large non-stick frying pan on a low heat and toast the pine nuts. When they are golden, add the butter to the pan with the remaining basil leaves. Finely grate in the lemon zest, stir and keep on a low heat.

Once the pan of water is boiling, add the gnudi. They only need a minute or two to cook, and will rise to the surface when ready. As soon as they rise, scoop them out of the pan with a slotted spoon straight into the basil butter. Remove the frying pan from the heat and toss everything together for 30 seconds, until glossy and shiny. Finish by finely grating over the reamining Parmesan and serve straight away.

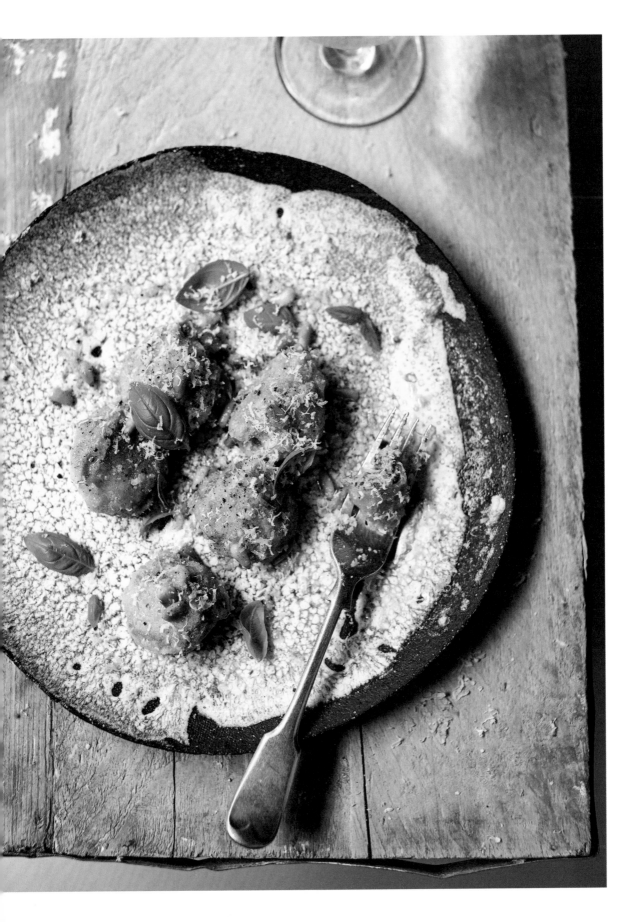

JERUSALEM ARTICHOKE AND THYME BARLEY RISOTTO

When I was a vegetarian I got lumbered with a lot of risottos and stuffed peppers over the years (we are talking many moons ago, and times have definitely improved for our non-carnivorous friends since then). Don't take me wrong, both are potentially beautiful things, but both are now dishes that make me shudder slightly. So when I first had risotto made with barley I was over the moon. Slightly nuttier than its rice counterpart, barley risotto is less creamy and more forgiving and the grains make for a much more interesting texture. I adore this dish, and feel free to use whatever is in season, switching the Jerusalem artichokes for celeriac, wild mushrooms or even parsnips.

SERVES 6

—

2 leeks

2 onions

350g Jerusalem artichokes

1.5 litres good vegetable stock

30g butter

olive oil

½ a bunch of thyme

300g pearl barley

80g strong hard cheese *(a mature Cheddar, Lincolnshire Poacher or Mrs Kirkham's Lancashire are perfect)*

2 heaped tablespoons crème fraîche

sea salt and freshly ground black pepper

½ a lemon

Trim, wash and finely slice the leeks. Peel and finely chop the onions. Peel the Jerusalem artichokes and cut into 1cm pieces. Heat the vegetable stock in a pan and keep it warm on the hob.

Place a wide casserole-style pan on a medium heat and add the butter and a little olive oil. Add the Jerusalem artichokes and fry for 8-10 minutes, until lightly golden all over. Add the leeks and onions and pick in the thyme leaves. Reduce the heat a little and sauté gently for around 15 minutes, until soft, sweet and sticky but not coloured. Stir in the pearl barley and 800ml of the stock and bring to the boil. Place the lid on the pan, reduce the heat to low and cook for around 30 minutes.

After the 30 minutes you want to start cooking the barley like a traditional risotto; lots of ladling in stock and stirring. Slowly ladle in the remaining hot stock and keep stirring for around 40 minutes, until it has all been absorbed and the barley is slightly creamy and cooked through. If the barley still has a bite, add a little more hot stock and stir and cook for a further 5–10 minutes.

When the risotto is ready, grate in the cheese and stir in the crème fraîche. Season to taste and finish by finely grating over the lemon zest.

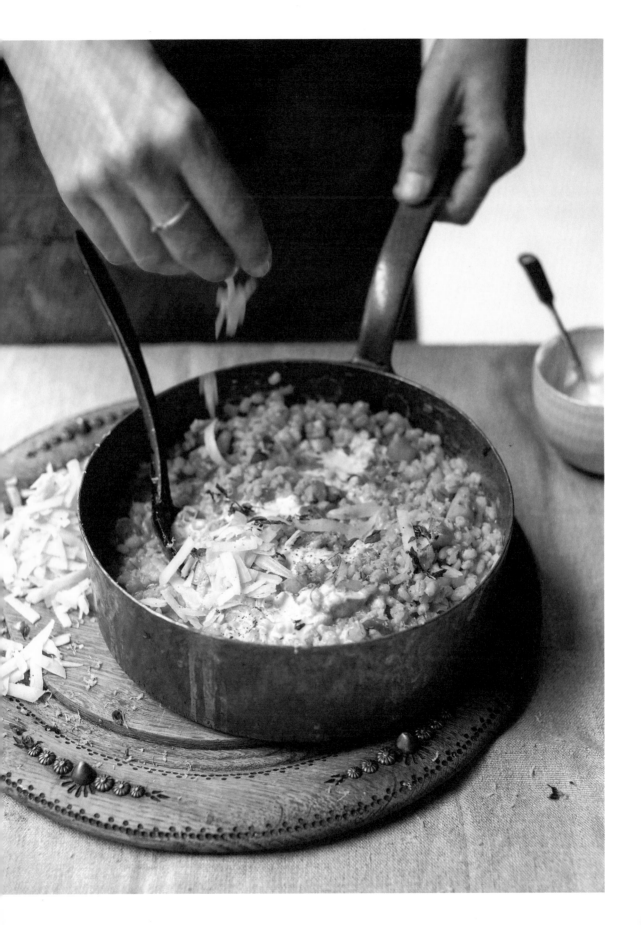

PORK AND PRAWN GYOZAS

My dear colleague Pete Begg (aka the food oracle) taught me how to make gyozas and I guarantee once you make these dreamy dumplings you'll be sold too. They are so easy, and the more practice you have the speedier you'll become. Once you're in the gyoza-making zone (and it's a wonderfully calming zone to be in), it's easy to make a whole load, so just freeze any extras – they make a perfect rainy-day lunch or snack.

MAKES 30

—

30 gyoza skins *(shop-bought or homemade - see below)*

½ a red chilli

2 garlic cloves

a 3cm piece of ginger

2 spring onions

150g white cabbage

150g pork mince

100g raw prawns, deveined

1 teaspoon sesame oil

½ tablespoon low-salt soy sauce

groundnut or vegetable oil

soy sauce, rice vinegar and sweet chilli oil, to serve *(or whatever you like!)*

TO MAKE YOUR OWN GYOZA SKINS

—

300g strong white bread flour

150ml boiling water

½ teaspoon salt

If making your own gyoza skins, follow the instructions on page 134. If using frozen gyoza skins, make sure they are defrosted before you use them – they only need about an hour out of the freezer. Either way, cover them with a slightly damp piece of kitchen paper to stop them drying out.

Deseed and roughly shop the chilli. Peel and roughly chop the garlic and ginger. Trim and chop the spring onions. Place them all in a food processor and blitz until finely chopped (alternatively you can do this by hand). Roughly chop the cabbage and add to the food processor with the pork, prawns, sesame oil and soy sauce, and blitz again until it is all chopped and you have a coarse paste. Scrape the mixture into a bowl. Alternatively just chop everything together by hand as finely as you can and mix. You don't have to use a food processor if you don't want to.

Making gyozas is really easy, and the more you make the quicker you'll get. Most important is to get your 'gyoza-making station' ready. You'll need your pork and prawn filling, the gyoza wrappers, a little bowl of cold water and a clean tray ready to line up the gyozas once they're made. Take one of the skins (keeping the pile covered with damp kitchen paper to keep them from drying out) and place it in the palm of your hand. Spoon a teaspoonful of the prawn mixture into the middle of the round (don't overfill the gyozas or you'll struggle to seal them), then damp the edge of the wrapper with a little water. Fold the wrapper in half and pleat the edges, pressing them down to seal completely. I fold the wrapper in half, pinch it in the middle and then pleat outwards one side, followed by the other. But anything goes, as long as they're well sealed. Keep going until you've used up all your filling. If it's taking you a while to get the hang of it, make sure to refrigerate any gyozas you've made to keep them from spoiling. »

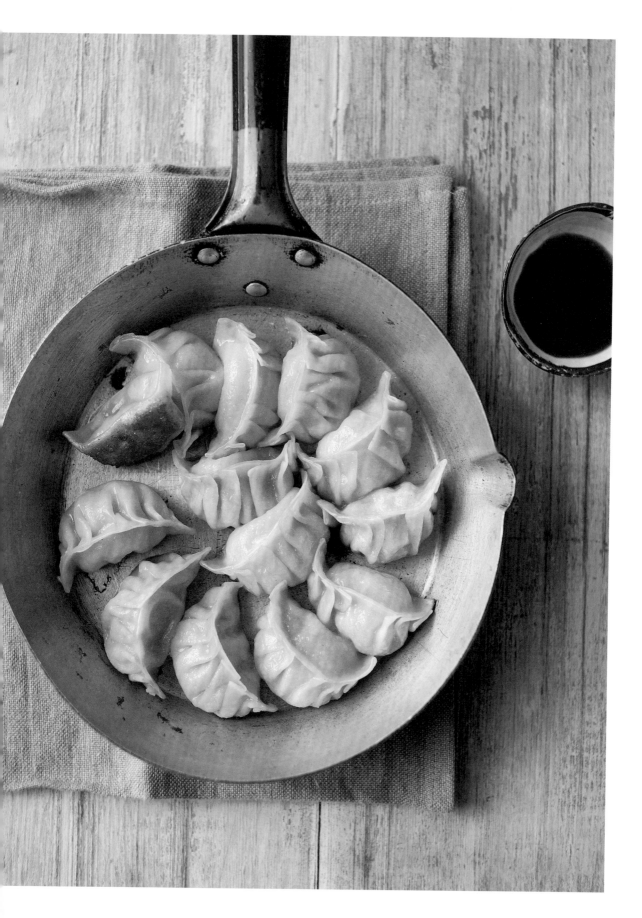

« Choose a non-stick frying pan or saucepan that is big enough to hold the amount of gyozas you want to cook in a single layer. Place it on a medium heat and drizzle in a tablespoon of groundnut or vegetable oil. As soon as it starts to get warm, place the gyozas in the pan, so that they are sitting upright, and fry them lightly so they start to turn golden underneath. As soon as they look a little crisp, after about 3 minutes, pour in enough water to come halfway up the side of the gyozas. Turn the heat up, bring to the boil, then cover with a lid. Reduce the heat to medium-low and cook for 8 minutes (you'll see the pink from the cooked prawns through the wrapper).

As soon as the gyozas are cooked, remove the lid and turn the heat up a little. The water should have almost completely evaporated and now you want the bottoms to get nice and crisp. Fry for a few more minutes, checking to make sure they don't burn, and serve. I like to serve them with soy sauce, chilli oil and rice vinegar, but you can use whatever you like.

TO MAKE YOUR OWN GYOZA SKINS
—

Mix the flour and salt together in a large bowl and stir in the 150ml of boiling water with a spoon. Keep stirring, adding a splash more water if it feels a little dry. As soon as the dough comes together and is cool enough to handle, start kneading with your hands. After 5 minutes you should have a nice smooth dough (and a nice clean bowl). Divide the dough evenly into 3, then each of those pieces into 2. You should end up with 6 evenly sized bits of dough. Roll each out into a sausage shape (this will make rolling out the skins later easier) and leave on a board, covered with a lightly damp tea towel, for 30 minutes to rest.

Once the dough has rested, cut one of the logs into 5 even pieces. Turn each nugget of dough on its side and roll into a round. Roll as evenly as you can, a little bigger than 8cm, then cut with an 8cm round pastry cutter to make it as even as possible (and discard the excess). Stack the pastry rounds and keep going with the dough logs until you've rolled them all out. You should end up with 30 gyoza skins.

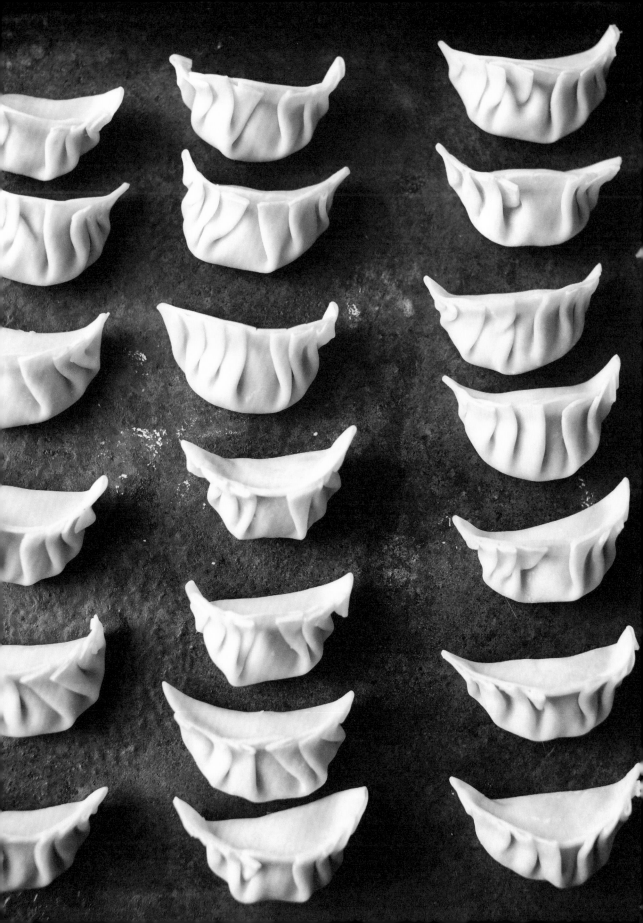

HEARTY FISH STEW WITH ALMOND SKORDALIA

This recipe is wonderfully balanced and manages to be hearty and indulgent, yet delicate at the same time. The key is in the base; take the time to sauté the veg slowly, and reduce the wine to give it the depth it needs, before adding the fish at the end.

SERVES 4
—

1 onion

5 garlic cloves

2 sticks of celery

1 bulb of fennel

1 bunch of flat-leaf parsley

a good pinch of saffron

Extra virgin olive oil

1 tablespoon fennel seeds

½ teaspoon dried chilli flakes

1 tablespoon tomato purée

175ml dry white wine

2 fresh bay leaves

1 litre good-quality fish stock

1 x 400g tin of plum tomatoes

sea salt and freshly ground black
   pepper

125g fregola or risotto rice

1 thick slice of good white bread,
   around 150g

50g almonds or walnuts

2 lemons

250g sea bass or bream fillets,
   skin on, scaled and pin-boned

300g monkfish or other firm white
   fish, trimmed

200g squid, cleaned

Peel the onion and 2 of the garlic cloves and chop finely. Trim and finely chop the celery and the fennel, reserving any fennel fronds for serving. Pick the parsley leaves and leave to one side, and finely slice the stalks. Put the saffron into a small bowl, cover with 50ml of boiling water and leave to one side.

Place a large casserole or stew-pot on a medium-low heat and pour in a good drizzle of olive oil. Add the chopped veg and and parsley stalks and sauté for 15 minutes, until softened but not coloured. Crush the fennel seeds in a mortar and pestle until finely ground, then add to the pan along with the chilli flakes and tomato purée, and fry for a couple more minutes. Add the wine to the pan along with the bay leaves and gently bring to the boil. Keep on a rolling boil for 5–8 minutes, until reduced by half, then add the fish stock, saffron water and tinned tomatoes. Season, turn up the heat and bring to the boil. As it starts to bubble, reduce the heat and cover with a lid. Simmer for around 30 minutes, then blitz a little with a stick blender. You don't have to do this, you can leave it as a chunky stew, but I like mine a little creamy too.

Add the fregola or rice to the pan, bring back to the boil, then leave to simmer for another 30 minutes uncovered, adding boiling water if it looks like it's thickening too much.

While the stew is ticking away, make the skordalia and prepare the fish. Trim the crusts off the bread and tear into small pieces. Blitz in a food processor until you have breadcrumbs, then spoon into a bowl. Peel and roughly chop the remaining 3 garlic cloves, pop them into the food processor with the almonds, half the parsley leaves and a good pinch of salt, and blitz until finely ground. Put the breadcrumbs back into the processor with 125ml of water and blitz while slowly pouring in enough extra virgin olive oil to give you a creamy texture, around 4-5 tablespoons. Squeeze in the juice of half of a lemon and season to taste. »

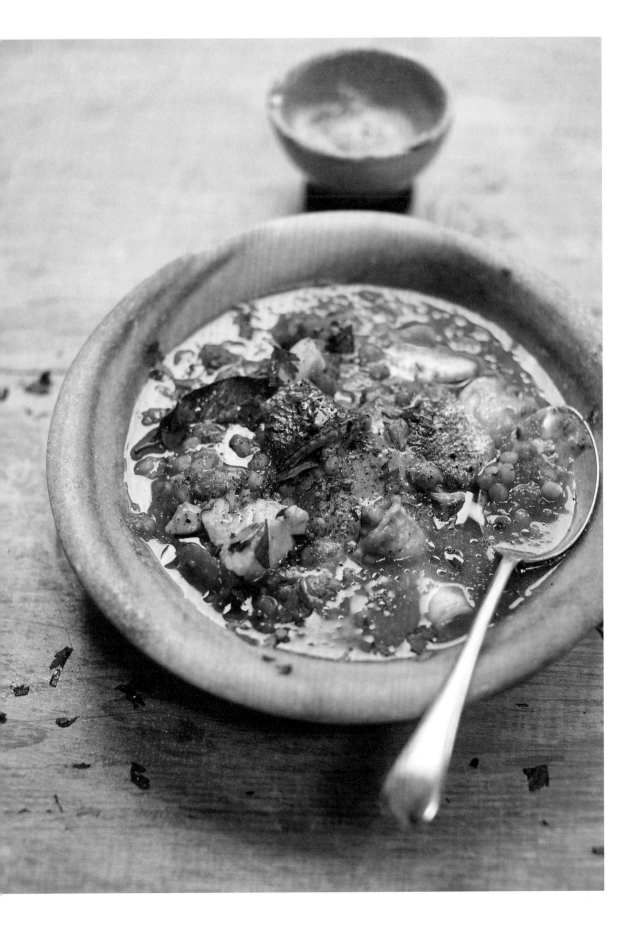

« Cut the fish and squid into 2½cm pieces, and when the stew has had 30 minutes, pop them on top. I like to poke the squid into the stew, along with the monkfish, and lay the sea bass on top. Cover with the lid and leave to poach for 10 minutes, until the fish is tender and just cooked through.

Finely chop the remaining parsley leaves and stir through the stew along with the juice of the remaining lemons. Check the seasoning and serve, ladled into bowls and topped with a spoonful of almond skordalia and any reserved fennel fronds (and a chunk of fresh bread on the side).

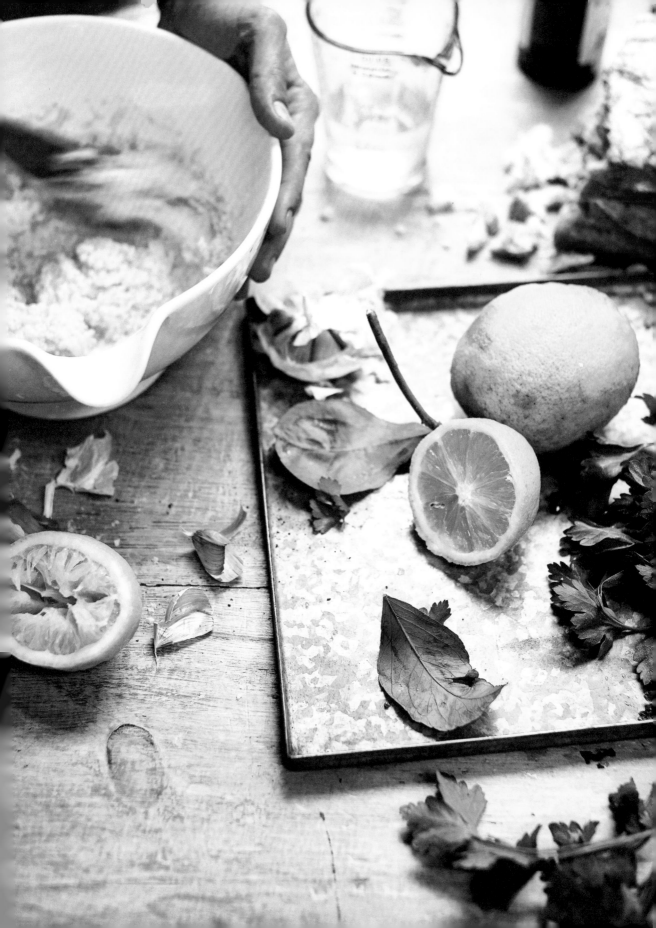

SLOW-COOKED CHICKEN RENDANG WITH GENTLY SPICED RICE

I'm not in the habit of substituting red meat with chicken – however, it really works here and makes for a slightly lighter version of an incredibly hearty meal. It's straightforward to make, too; once you've made the paste there isn't a lot to do other than stir and watch. You want the chicken to be sticky and gnarly, but don't leave it unattended or it'll catch.

SERVES 6
—

300g basmati rice

sea salt and freshly ground black
    pepper

a 2cm piece of ginger

4 garlic cloves

4 shallots

1 teaspoon turmeric

1 ½ tablespoons dried chilli flakes

2 sticks of lemongrass

a 2cm piece of galangal *(if you
    can't find galangal, use extra
    ginger)*

groundnut or vegetable oil

1 star anise

1 x 400g tin of coconut milk

4 kaffir lime leaves

1kg chicken thighs, boneless and
    skinless

1 tablespoon soft light brown
    sugar

75g desiccated coconut (ideally
    unsweetened)

a knob of butter

1 cinnamon stick

nutmeg

If you can bear it, cook your rice the day before, or well in advance. Cold cooked rice is easier to stir-fry and flavour. Fill a large saucepan with water, add a generous pinch of salt and place on a high heat. Rinse the rice in a sieve, under cold running water, then spoon into the boiling water. Reduce the heat to medium-low, so it is gently bubbling away, and cook for around 9 minutes, or according to the packet instructions. When the rice is just ready, drain it, rinse under cold water again and spread it out on a tray to cool. Transfer to a bowl and refrigerate until needed.

Peel and roughly chop the ginger, 2 garlic cloves and the shallots. Put into a food processor with the turmeric and chilli flakes. Add a splash of water and blitz the spices to a paste. Trim the lemongrass and bash them gently in a mortar and pestle. Peel and finely chop the galangal.

Put a large casserole-type pan on a medium heat and pour in a glug of groundnut or vegetable oil. Add the star anise and lemongrass and fry for a minute. Spoon in all the spice paste from the food processor and the chopped galangal, and reduce the heat a little. Gently sauté for 12–15 minutes to soften, stirring often so it doesn't catch. Add the coconut milk to the pan along with the kaffir lime leaves, then turn the heat up a little and gently bring to the boil.

Chop the chicken into large pieces and add to the pan. Stir in the brown sugar and a good pinch of salt and pepper. Bring to the boil, then cover the pan and cook on the lowest heat for around 40 minutes.

While the chicken is cooking, toast the coconut. If your desiccated coconut is sweetened, soak it in a small bowl in boiling water for a few minutes, then drain it in a sieve to remove the excess sugar. Toast the coconut in a dry frying pan over a low heat until lightly golden, then keep to one side.

When the chicken is ready, remove the lid and stir in the toasted coconut. Turn up the heat and bring the rendang back to the boil. You want to cook it over a medium-high heat for a further 35-40 minutes, so that the liquid completely cooks away and you are left with sticky and gnarly chicken, coated in the coconut spice mix.

For the rice, place a large frying pan on a medium heat and add the knob of butter with a slight drizzle of groundnut or vegetable oil. Peel and finely slice the remaining 2 garlic cloves and add to the pan along with the cinnamon stick. Fry for a couple of minutes, until golden, then add the cold cooked rice to the pan. Finely grate over a quarter of the nutmeg, season the rice generously and fry for 5–7 minutes, stirring often, until piping hot throughout. Serve alongside the chicken rendang, with a bowl of steamed beans or greens.

ROAST HARISSA BUTTER CHICKEN AND CRACKED WHEAT

This is a perfect Sunday dinner if you want something a little different but still really special. Once you've cooked your chicken this way I guarantee you'll be converted, and any leftover buttery chicken is epic in a sandwich the next day.

SERVES 4

—

4 garlic cloves

1 preserved lemon

1 teaspoon cumin seeds

1 teaspoon coriander seeds

1 teaspoon sweet smoked paprika

2 tablespoons harissa

a bunch of coriander

a bunch of parsley

sea salt and freshly ground black
  pepper

80g butter, at room temperature

olive oil

1 x 1.6kg chicken

1 lemon

425ml fresh chicken stock

1 onion

2 tomatoes

350g bulgur wheat

Greek yoghurt, to serve

Preheat your oven to 190°C/gas 5. Peel the garlic. Halve the preserved lemon and remove the seeds. In a dry frying pan toast the cumin and coriander seeds until lightly toasted. Place in a food processor along with the paprika, preserved lemon, harissa, half the coriander and parsley (stalks and all) and the garlic. Season well and blitz to a paste. Add the butter and 2 tablespoons of olive oil and pulse until smooth.

Use your hands to carefully prise the chicken skin away from each breast, to create a pocket. Slash the skin on the thighs and rub the butter all over – under the skin mainly and all over the top. Halve the lemon and pop it into the chicken cavity, then place in a small snug-fitting roasting tray. Put it into the oven and roast for around 1¼ hours, or until golden and crisp but cooked through – check that the juices run clear around the thigh area. Baste the chicken a couple of times during cooking with the buttery juices in the tray.

When the chicken has about 20 minutes left to cook, start the bulgur wheat. Heat your chicken stock in a medium pan. Meanwhile peel and finely chop the onion, and deseed and finely chop the tomatoes. Pour a glug of olive oil into a saucepan and put on a medium-low heat. Add the onion and sauté for 10 minutes, until soft. Add the tomatoes and cook for a further 5 minutes, then add the bulgur wheat. Stir for a minute, then add the hot chicken stock and season lightly. Bring to the boil, pop on the lid, then reduce the heat to low. Simmer for 8 minutes, until the wheat is cooked through and fluffy, then remove from the heat. Cover the pan with a tea towel and put a lid on top to keep it warm. Chop the rest of the coriander and parsley leaves and stir through the bulgur wheat.

When the chicken is ready, leave to rest for 10 minutes, then squeeze over the lemon from the cavity and carve it up – you can carve traditionally or shred the meat into the buttery juices to keep the meat insanely moist. Serve with the bulgur wheat and tangy thick Greek yoghurt.

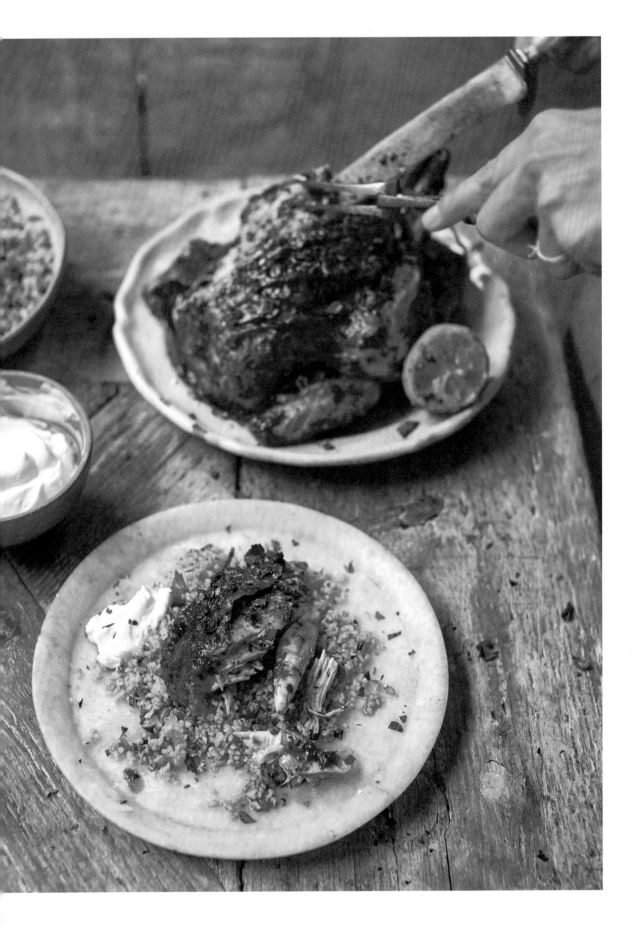

HAM HOCKS, FENNEL AND BEANS

This is my ideal way of cooking: little prep, hours in the oven and a delicious and comforting result. And if you can bear it, make sure there are leftovers, as it's even better the next day.

SERVES 6-8
—

400g dried borlotti, flageolet or cannellini beans

2 gammon hocks, around 750g each, skin removed *(get your butcher to do this for you)*

1½ tablespoons fennel seeds

1 teaspoon dried chilli flakes

1 whole bulb of garlic

sea salt and freshly ground black pepper

a few sprigs of rosemary and thyme

olive oil

2 bulbs of fennel

2 fresh bay leaves

175ml white wine

a splash of white wine vinegar

½ a bunch of flat-leaf parsley

Make sure you remember to start this dish the night before. You'll need to soak the beans in plenty of cold water to soften them, and soak the ham hocks to get rid of all the excess salt, leaving them overnight in the fridge.

Preheat your oven to 170°C/gas 3.

In a mortar and pestle, bash the fennel seeds and chilli flakes to a coarse powder. Peel 4 of the garlic cloves and add, along with a good pinch of salt. Pick the rosemary and thyme leaves and add to the mortar, then bash everything together until you have a thick paste. Muddle in a couple of tablespoons of olive oil to loosen, then, using a paring knife, slice a few pockets in the ham hocks and rub the paste all over. Leave to one side.

Trim the fennel bulbs and cut them into wedges about 2cm thick, then place in a large casserole dish or ovenproof saucepan. Add the drained soaked beans, bay leaves, remaining unpeeled garlic cloves and wine. Place the pot on a high heat and bring the wine to the boil, then cook it rapidly for 4-5 minutes, until almost all the wine is cooked away. Add enough water to just cover the beans and bring everything to the boil. Pop the coated ham hocks (and any leftover garlic herb rub) into the dish and cover with the lid. Place in the preheated oven for around 4 hours, or until the ham is tender and pulls away from the bone. Baste the meat a couple of times during cooking, and add a splash of boiling water if it looks like the beans are drying out – you want them to be creamy and soft.

When the pork is cooked, remove the lid and drizzle with a little olive oil, then pop the pot back into the oven uncovered. Turn the heat up to 200°C/gas 6 and cook for a further 20 minutes, so the hocks get a little crispy. When they're ready, finish the beans with a splash of white wine vinegar and season to taste. Pick and chop the parsley leaves and stir through the beans. I like to shred the meat into the beans and serve, or alternatively transfer it to a platter and let everyone dig in.

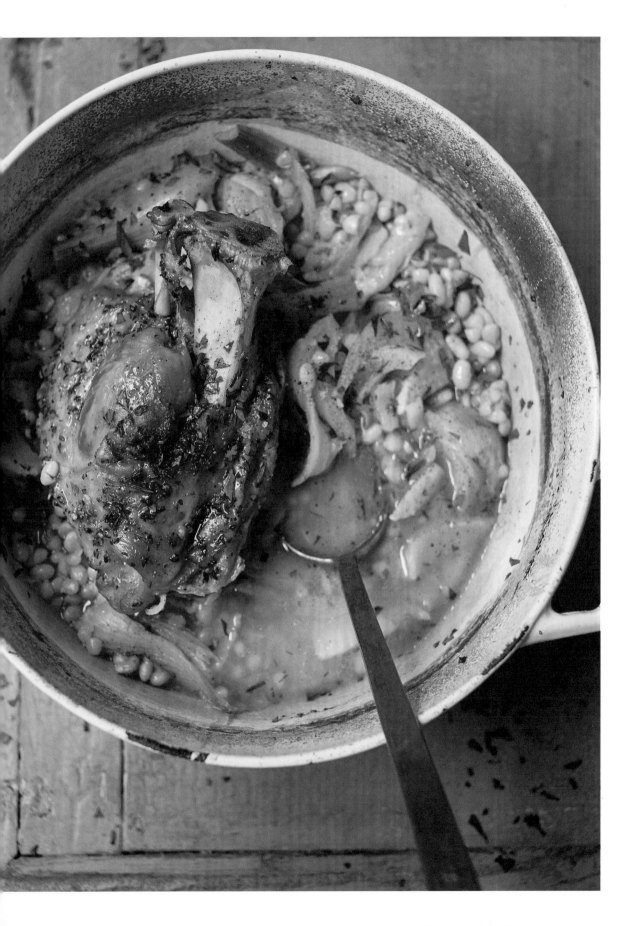

STICKY PORK BELLY SALAD WITH FENNEL AND CHILLI

Don't let the slightly long ingredients list put you off with this one, it's absolutely delicious and a fantastic way of using a slow-cook cut of meat in a lighter way. If you are short of time, poach the pork belly the day before. It'll sit happily in the broth overnight (covered in the fridge, of course).

SERVES 4

—

600ml beef stock

100g soft dark brown sugar

1 star anise

1 teaspoon Chinese five-spice

3 tablespoons white wine vinegar

3 tablespoons fish sauce

1 garlic clove

1 stick of lemongrass

700g pork belly, skinless and boneless

1 red chilli

1 lime

½ tablespoon honey

1 tablespoon sesame oil

1 tablespoon groundnut oil

a bunch of mint

½ a bunch of dill

30g toasted peanuts

1 chicory

70g watercress

2 bulbs of fennel

4 spring onions

Pour the stock into a large saucepan and stir in 60g of the sugar along with the star anise, five-spice, white wine vinegar and 2 tablespoons of the fish sauce. Crush the garlic clove and lemongrass and add to the pan, then place on a medium heat. Gently bring to the boil, then carefully add the pork belly. Once the stock starts to bubble, reduce the heat to low and leave to tick away for 1 hour, until the belly is cooked through and tender but still holding its shape. If the stock runs low, top it up with boiling water to keep the meat covered during cooking. Turn off the heat and leave the pork to cool in the broth for around 20 minutes.

While the pork is cooling, make the dressing and prepare the rest of the salad. Deseed and finely chop the chilli and pop into a small bowl. Squeeze in the juice of the lime, then add the honey, sesame oil, groundnut oil and the remaining 1 tablespoon of fish sauce. Whisk together and leave to one side. Pick and roughly chop the mint and dill leaves, and roughly chop the peanuts. Roughly chop the chicory, then wash and spin along with the watercress. Trim and slice the fennel into thin shavings, using a mandolin or a potato peeler, and pop them into a bowl of cold water with a few ice cubes – this will make the shavings crisp. Trim and finely slice the spring onions, into strips if you can, but rounds is fine too.

When you are ready to assemble your salad, preheat your grill to medium high. Remove the pork from the broth and cut it into 1cm slices. Lay them out on a roasting tray and sprinkle with the remaining 40g of sugar. Grill the pork for around 5–10 minutes, until sticky and caramelised. Place most of the pork slices erratically on a large platter. Drain and spin dry the fennel and mix in a large bowl with the salad leaves, herbs, spring onions and dressing. Scatter the salad over the platter and top with the remaining pork slices. Finish by sprinkling over the chopped peanuts.

—

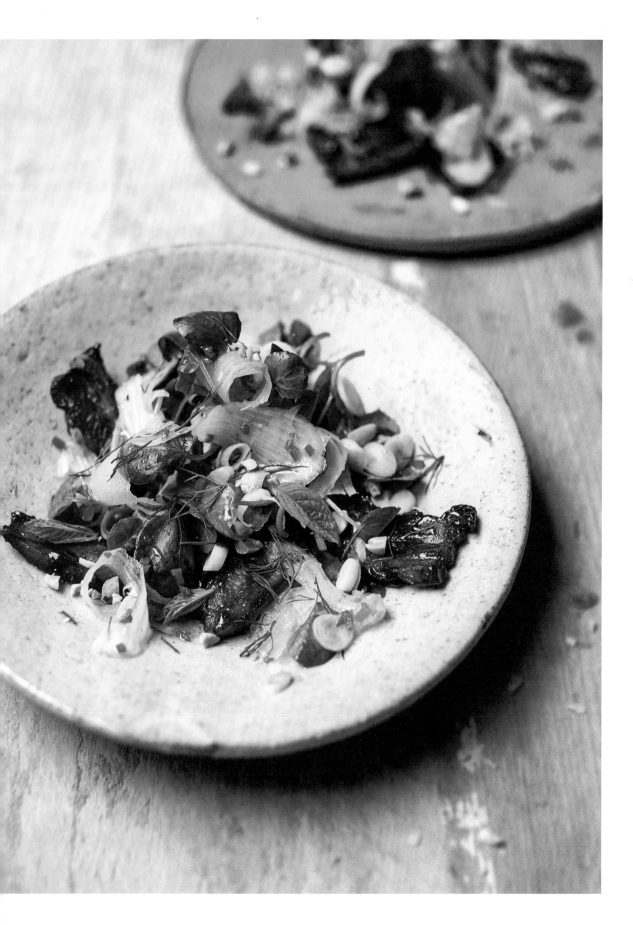

PECAN AND SAUSAGE STUFFING MAC 'N' CHEESE

There's been a real mac 'n' cheese resurgence recently, with it popping up on menus all over. And I do love it, it's pure nostalgia. Some like it crazy cheesy, some super sloppy – it's a personal thing. This is my favourite way of making it. Cheesy, oozy, with nuggets of sausage and ham laced throughout. It's so naughty, but so good.

SERVES 6-8

—

sea salt and freshly ground black pepper

4 garlic cloves

75g butter

100g plain flour

2 teaspoons English mustard

1.3 litres full-fat or semi-skimmed milk

200g mature Cheddar

500g macaroni

100g cooked/leftover ham

200g leftover cooked sausage stuffing *(if you haven't got any leftovers don't worry, just use the cooked meat from good-quality sausages)*

1 tablespoon maple syrup

a few sprigs of rosemary

olive oil

30g pecans

Preheat the oven to 180°C/gas 4. Bring a large pan of well-salted water to the boil.

Peel and finely slice the garlic. Melt the butter in a large saucepan over a medium-low heat, then add the garlic and the flour and keep stirring until you have a caramel-coloured roux. Stir in the mustard, then slowly add the milk, whisking it in as you go so the sauce is as creamy and smooth as possible. Keep adding and whisking until all the milk has been added. Very gently bring the sauce to a simmer, then cook over a low heat for 5 minutes until thickened and smooth. Coarsely grate in most of the Cheddar, stir it in, then season to taste.

While the sauce is ticking away, cook the pasta a couple of minutes less than the packet instructions, and drain, reserving a large mugful (300ml) of the pasta water. Chop and shred the ham and stuffing, so it is all roughly 1cm in size, and place in a medium-size non-stick frying pan over a medium-low heat and glaze with the maple syrup. Fry until golden and sticky.

When you are ready to bake your mac 'n' cheese, pour the cooked macaroni into the cheese sauce and mix. Add all the reserved pasta water and keep stirring. It might feel loose, but the pasta will carry on cooking and the sauce will thicken up in the oven. Stir in most of the ham and stuffing and pour the mixture into a large ovenproof baking dish. Grate over the remaining cheese and scatter over the remaining meat.

Pick the rosemary leaves and toss with a little olive oil. Chop the pecans and add to the rosemary. Sprinkle over the top of the dish and pop it into the oven. Bake for 25–30 minutes, until golden on top and bubbling. Leave it to sit for a couple of minutes, then serve, with a crisp green salad.

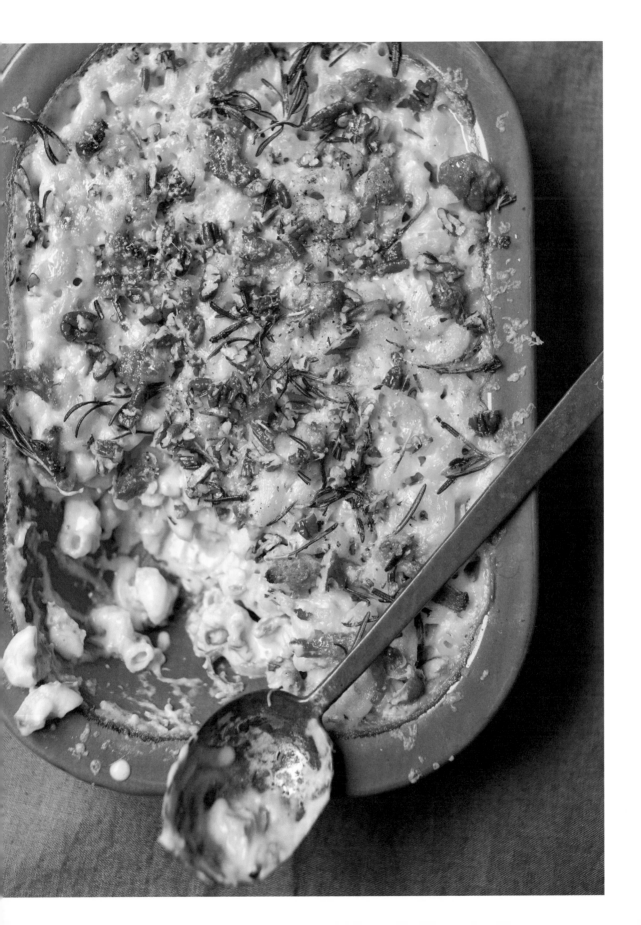

LANCASHIRE PIE BARM

A dedication to Pete, my pie-loving husband, this is slow and gentle cooking at its best. Slow-cooked beef shin, enrobed in suet pastry – it's a firm family favourite. You could serve these beauties with mash and gravy for a traditional dinner, but if you're really brave, serve the pies in a buttered barm cake with copious amounts of brown sauce – just like he does.

MAKES 4 PIES

—

1 onion

1 carrot

olive oil

2 fresh bay leaves

250g beef shin

525g plain flour

sea salt and freshly ground black
     pepper

1 teaspoon English mustard

1 tablespoon Worcestershire sauce

250ml beef stock

250g suet or cold butter

150g Maris Piper potatoes

butter, for greasing

50g mature Cheddar

a splash of milk

4 barm cakes or baps, buttered
     (optional)

brown sauce, to serve

Peel and finely chop the onion and carrot. Heat a good drizzle of olive oil in a large saucepan over a medium-low heat. Add the onion, carrot and bay leaves and sauté for 10 minutes, until soft but not browned.

Cut the beef into 2½cm chunks removing any excess fat and toss with 25g of the flour and a little pinch of salt and pepper, until coated. When the onion and carrot are ready, spoon them into a bowl, then add another drizzle of oil to the pan and fry the beef for 5 minutes, until browned. Return the softened onion and carrot to the pan, along with the mustard and Worcestershire sauce, and fry for a further 1–2 minutes, until everything is thoroughly mixed.

Add the stock, gently bring to the boil, then simmer, lid on, over a low heat for 2 hours, stirring occasionally, until the meat is soft and tender.

Meanwhile make the pastry. In a bowl mix together the suet (or coarsely grate in the butter) and the rest of the flour with a little salt and pepper. Using your hands, mix in 100ml of cold water and bring it together until it forms a dough. Wrap in clingfilm and chill in the fridge for at least 20 minutes.

Peel the potatoes and cut into 2½cm chunks. Put a large saucepan of water on to boil, and boil the potatoes for 10–12 minutes until just cooked. Drain in a colander and leave to steam dry completely.

When the beef filling is ready, take the pan off the heat, remove the bay leaves and stir in the potatoes. Leave to cool for 10 minutes, or, if you're making it in advance, leave to cool completely and refrigerate until you are ready. (If you have time, it's almost easier making the filling in advance.) »

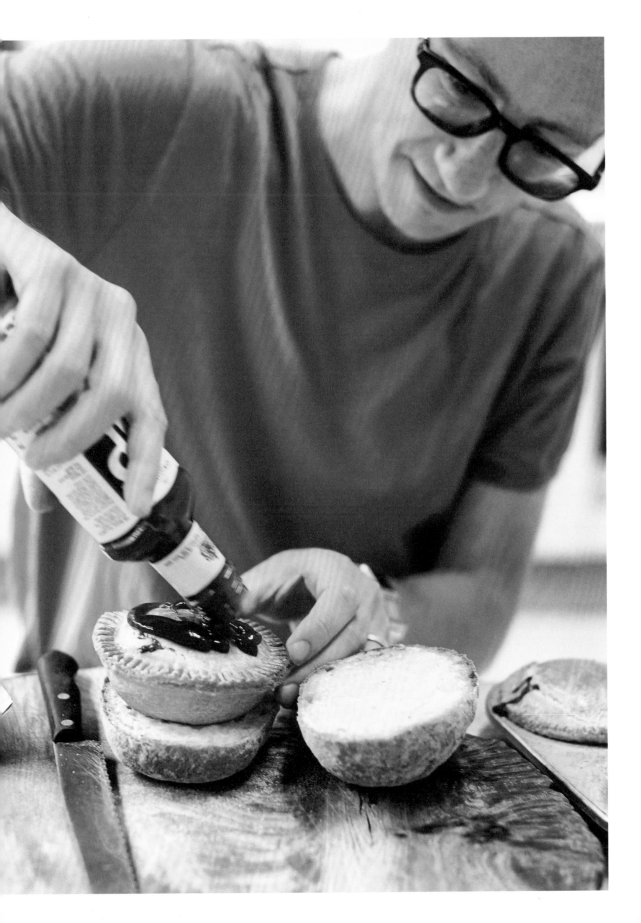

« To build your pies, preheat the oven to 180°C/gas 4. Take the pastry out of the fridge and divide into 8. Grease four 12cm pie tins, then roll out 4 pieces of the dough into a circle larger than the tins, about ½cm thick. Line each tin with a rolled-out piece of dough, pushing it into the edges, then trim off the excess. Fill each one with a quarter of the filling, crumble a quarter of the Cheddar on top and push it into the meat a little. Roll out the extra balls of dough, so they are a little larger than the pie, and drape them on top. Press the edges of the pastry together, and crimp to seal.

Snip a little hole in the pastry top of each pie to let steam escape, then brush with milk. Place them on a baking sheet and bake in the bottom of the oven for 50 minutes–1 hour, or until golden and crisp.

Leave the pies to cool in the tins for 10 minutes, then gently remove. Eat however you like, but ideally in a freshly buttered barm cake, with a good squeeze of brown sauce inside.

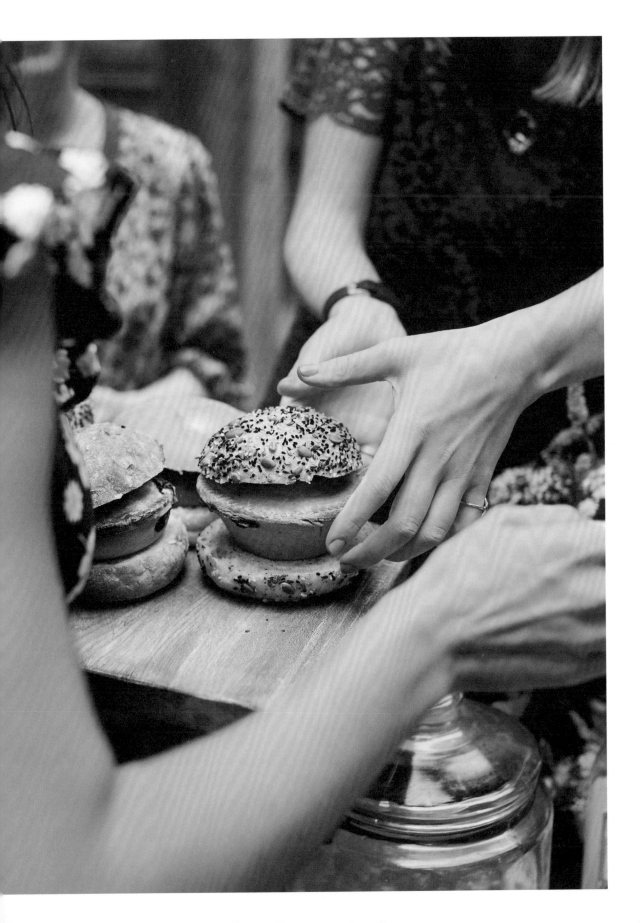

ADOBO BRISKET WITH GRIDDLED PINEAPPLE SALSA

The flavours in this marinade are heavily influenced by our favourite meal on a recent trip to Mexico; slow-cooked beef- and pork-filled tacos, on the side of a road. So good was this family's truck that we were advised to get there around 11 a.m. if we didn't want to miss out, and it was so worth it. Punchy but not spicy, this beef brisket dish is perfect for a dinner, even for a party. Serve this tender shreddable brisket with the salsa, a stack of tacos or tortillas, and let people dig in.

SERVES 8

—

4 dried ancho chillies

1 tablespoon cumin seeds

6 garlic cloves

2 shallots

½ teaspoon ground cloves

1 tablespoon dried chilli flakes

1 tablespoon dried oregano

1 orange

25g cacao (optional)

2 tablespoons red wine vinegar

sea salt and freshly ground black pepper

1.4kg beef brisket, boned and rolled

olive oil

2 cinnamon sticks

2 fresh bay leaves

500ml beef stock

1 red onion

1 red chilli

2 limes

½ a ripe pineapple

½ a bunch of coriander

rice and tortillas, to serve

Preheat the oven to 180°C/gas 4. Put the ancho chillies on a small baking tray and place in the oven for 2–3 minutes, until lightly toasted. Transfer them to a small saucepan and add enough water to just cover. Place the pan on a medium heat and gently bring to the boil. Remove from the heat and leave the chillies and liquid to cool completely.

Dry toast the cumin seeds in a small pan over a low heat, until they start smelling wonderful. When the chillies are cold, remove and discard their stalks (reserving the liquid) and put them into a blender. Peel the garlic and shallots and roughly chop, adding them to the blender also. Add the ground cloves, toasted cumin seeds, chilli flakes and oregano, then finely grate in the orange zest and squeeze in the juice, and grate in the cacao if using. Add 1 tablespoon of the red wine vinegar, season well and add a splash of the chilli soaking water. Blitz until you have a thick paste, adding more of the chilli water if it is too thick. Spoon the chilli paste into a large bowl and add the brisket. Spread the paste all over, so the meat is completely covered, and leave to marinate in the fridge for a few hours, or overnight if possible.

When you are ready to cook the brisket, place a casserole style pan, one that will hold the brisket pretty snugly, on a medium heat and preheat the oven to 140°C/gas 1. Pour a good glug of oil into the pan and add the marinated beef, browning it on all sides. When it has browned, add the cinnamon and bay leaves to the pan along with any remaining marinade and pour in enough beef stock to come just over halfway up the meat. Turn the heat to high, and as soon as it starts to boil, remove from the heat.

Tear a piece of greaseproof paper, slightly bigger than the pan, and rinse under the tap. Squeeze out the excess water, then tuck the damp paper »

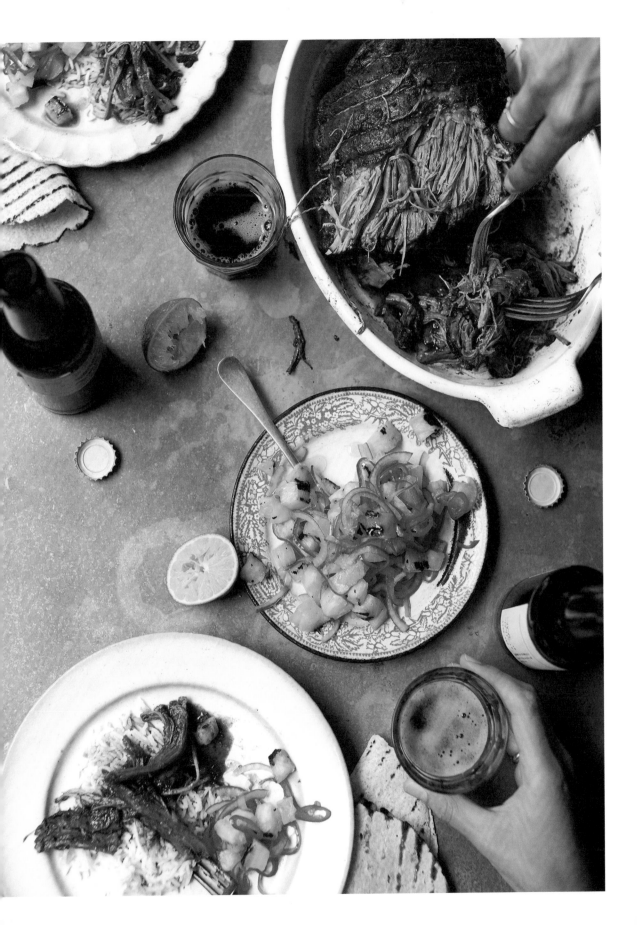

« over the top of the brisket. Cover with the lid and pop the dish into the oven. Cook for 3½–4 hours, until the meat is tender and shreds easily. Check it twice during cooking, turning it over so it all gets basted, and topping up the liquid if it starts to look a little dry.

While the brisket is cooking, make the salsa. Finely slice the red onion and chilli – deseeding if you don't want it too hot. Transfer to a bowl, squeeze in the juice of both limes and stir in the remaining 1 tablespoon of red wine vinegar. Leave to one side for 30 minutes. Pop a griddle pan on a high heat. Trim the pineapple half, remove the skin and cut into quarters lengthways. Remove the core, and pop the wedges on to the hot griddle. Keep turning the pineapple, giving it a few minutes on all sides, so it is charred all over. Remove from the griddle, leave to cool, then chop into small pieces, around 1cm big. Pick and chop the coriander leaves also, and pop everything into the bowl with the lime-dressed red onion. Toss together well and season to taste.

When the brisket is ready, remove the meat from the pot and leave on a board to rest for 15 minutes. Place the pan on the hob and boil the adobo sauce over a high heat, until reduced and thickened – you want a dense, dark gravy to dress the brisket. Transfer the meat back to the casserole dish or to a serving dish, untie the string, and pour over the thickened adobo sauce. Shred the meat with two forks and serve alongside the pineapple salsa. Perfect with steamed rice and griddled tortillas.

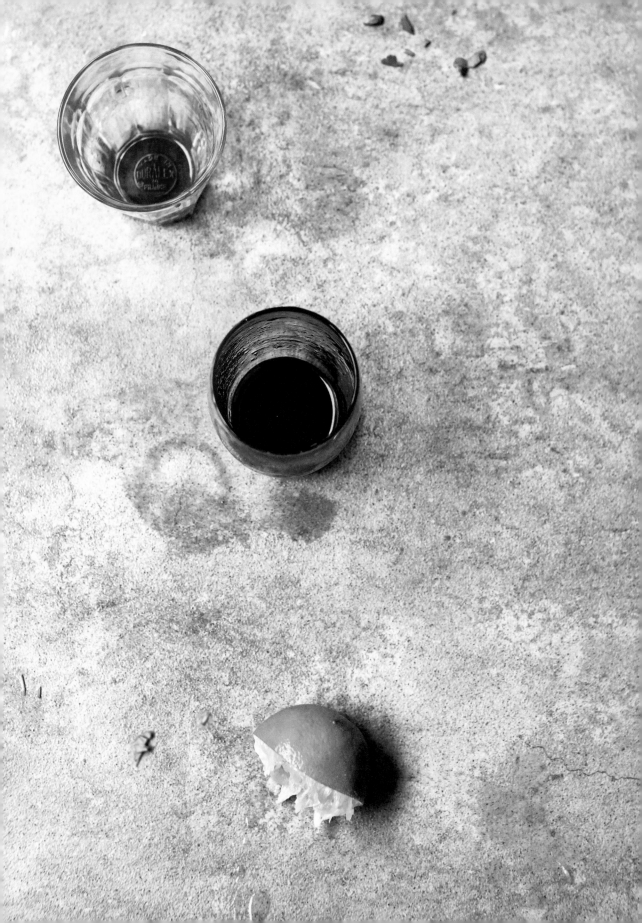

SPICED LAMB WITH DATES AND HERB-DRESSED FARRO

I made this recipe recently for my yiayia, as she hadn't been very well, and I wanted to make sure she was getting some rest while keeping her strength up. It feels like the perfect comforting get-well dish, full of warming spices, without being spicy.

SERVES 6
—

2 red onions

4 garlic cloves

2 sticks of celery

olive oil

800g lamb neck fillet

4 medjool dates

1 teaspoon ground coriander

1 teaspoon ground cumin

½ tablespoon ras el hanout

1 orange

1 x 400g tin of plum tomatoes

350ml chicken stock

75g red lentils

sea salt and freshly ground black
  pepper

FOR THE FARRO
—

1 onion

2 garlic cloves

a large knob of butter

1 cinnamon stick

300g farro

1 litre boiling water

½ a bunch of coriander

½ a bunch of mint

Greek yoghurt, to serve

Preheat your oven to 170°C/gas 3. Peel and finely slice the onions and garlic and finely slice the celery. Place a large casserole-style pan or ovenproof saucepan on a medium-low heat and pour in a glug of olive oil. Add the sliced veg and sauté for around 10 minutes, until everything is soft and sticky, but not coloured.

While the veg are cooking, cut the lamb into 2½cm chunks. Remove the stones from the dates, then chop them as finely as you can. When the veg are ready, add the ground coriander, ground cumin and ras el hanout to the pan and fry for about a minute, then add the meat. Turn the heat up a little and fry the meat for around 5–10 minutes, until it is browned all over. Add the chopped dates to the pan, finely grate in the zest of half of the orange, and squeeze in all the juice. Add the tinned tomatoes and chicken stock and gently bring everything to the boil. Once it starts to bubble, remove from the heat and pop a lid on the pot. Place it in the oven for an hour, so that the meat is on its way to being deliciously tender, then take it out and stir in the red lentils. Cover with the lid, put back into the oven and cook for a further hour, until the meat is falling apart and the stew is deliciously thick. Season to taste.

Once the lentils have been stirred through the stew, start making the farro. Peel and finely chop the onion and garlic. Melt the butter in a large saucepan over a medium-low heat and add the chopped veg. Sauté for 12–15 minutes, until soft and sticky, then add the cinnamon and farro. Stir for a minute, then add the litre of boiling water and season well. Bring to the boil, then reduce the heat to low, cover the pan and simmer for 15 minutes, until cooked perfectly.

Pick the coriander and mint leaves, discarding the stalks, and finely chop. Stir through the farro just before serving. Serve alongside the slow-cooked lamb with a pile of flatbreads and some thick tangy Greek yoghurt.

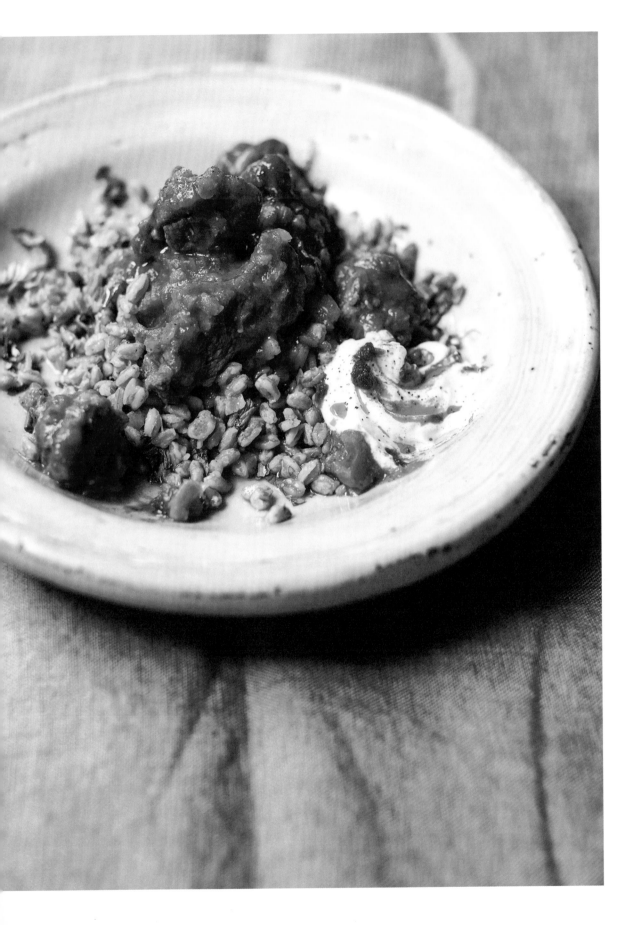

CINNAMON-BRAISED LAMB SHANKS

Slow-cooked and tender, these shanks are rich, warming and fragrant. They are perfect for entertaining, as they need little attention, or just if you fancy a change to your Sunday roast. Also cinnamon is believed to be full of health benefits, including cholesterol-reducing and anti-inflammatory properties.

SERVES 4

—

4 garlic cloves

a 4cm piece of ginger

100g golden raisins

1 tablespoon ground cinnamon

2 red chillies

2 teaspoons ground coriander

200ml natural yoghurt

sea salt and freshly ground black
   pepper

4 lamb shanks

8 shallots

groundnut or vegetable oil

1 cinnamon stick

2 star anise

1 fresh bay leaf

500ml chicken stock

Peel and roughly chop the garlic and ginger and blitz in a food processor with the raisins, ground cinnamon, chillies and ground coriander. Add the yoghurt, and a good pinch of salt and pepper, and pulse until just mixed. Make incisions in the lamb shanks and place in a bowl. Rub the marinade into the meat, then cover and marinate for a few hours, or even for a day if possible.

When you are ready to cook the meat, peel and finely slice the shallots. Pour a drizzle of groundnut or vegetable oil into a deep, heavy-based casserole – one large enough to hold all the shanks – and fry the cinnamon stick, star anise and bay leaf for a minute. Add the shallots, then turn the heat right down and sauté for 10 minutes, until soft and sticky. Spoon the mixture into a bowl and leave to one side.

Drizzle a little more oil into the casserole and turn up the heat. Brown the lamb shanks in batches, reserving any marinade left in the bowl. When the meat is brown on all sides, return it all to the pan with the softened shallots and any reserved marinade. Pour in the chicken stock and bring to the boil. Cover with a lid, then cook over a low heat for 3 hours, turning the shanks regularly and adding more stock if it gets too dry. The lamb should be tender and falling off the bone. Remove the shanks from the pan and cover with foil to keep warm. Turn up the heat and let the sauce bubble away for around 10 minutes, until thickened and rich.

Return the lamb shanks to the pot and serve. Perfect with mashed potato or creamed cauliflower and greens, or even steaming basmati rice.

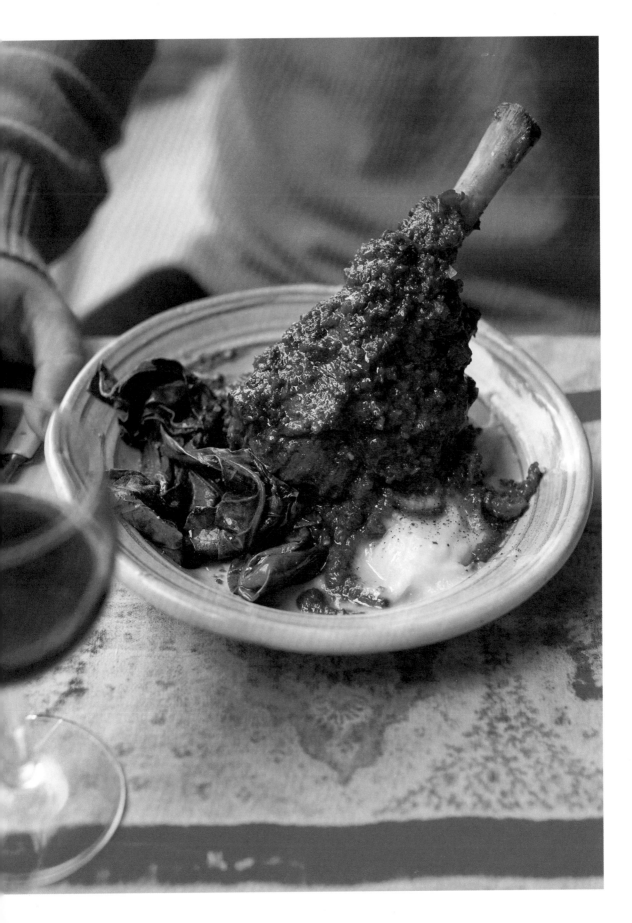

VENISON, WILD MUSHROOM AND CELERIAC TOPPED PIE

I felt pretty nervous presenting this beast of a pie to my right-hand woman, Isla, as she is a true Scotswoman, and married to Angus, a true Scotsman. However, their feedback was amazing, Angus devoured the lot, and that's good enough for me.

SERVES 8
—

1kg venison shoulder or neck fillet

1 tablespoon juniper berries

2 tablespoons plain flour

sea salt and freshly ground black pepper

½ a bunch of rosemary

500g wild mushrooms

2 garlic cloves

2 onions

2 sticks of celery

olive oil

2 fresh bay leaves

100ml sloe gin (*if you don't have it you can use a good ale*)

1 tablespoon Worcestershire sauce

400ml beef stock

2 tablespoons redcurrant jelly

1 large celeriac (around 650g)

800g Maris Piper potatoes

50g butter

a splash of milk

Cut the venison into 3–4 cm pieces. Crush the juniper berries in a mortar and pestle. Spoon into a bowl with the meat, sprinkle with the flour and a good pinch of salt and pepper, and toss to coat. Finely chop the rosemary leaves. Wipe the mushrooms clean and tear into bite-size pieces. Peel and finely slice the garlic and onions. Trim and slice the celery. Pour a good drizzle of oil into a large pan over a medium heat. Brown the meat, in batches if necessary, then set to one side. Put the pan back on a medium heat, add the garlic and the mushrooms and fry for a few minutes until they begin to soften, then add the onion, celery and rosemary and reduce the heat to low. Sauté for about 10 minutes, until softened, then return the meat to the pan.

Add the bay leaves and the sloe gin or ale, then bring to the boil and cook for a couple of minutes until reduced slightly. Stir in the Worcestershire sauce, and add enough beef stock to cover. Return to the boil, then reduce the heat to a simmer. Cover and cook gently for 2½–3 hours, or until the meat is incredibly tender and shreds easily, and the gravy is rich and thick. Finish by stirring in the redcurrant jelly, then season to taste.

When your meat is almost ready, preheat the oven to 180°C/gas 4. Peel the celeriac and potatoes and cut into even-size chunks. Place the potatoes in a large pan of salted water, bring to the boil, and cook for around 10–15 minutes, until cooked through. Drain and steam dry. At the same time do the same with the celeriac, but cook it for around 8–10 minutes. When all the veg are ready, mash with the butter and a splash of milk, then season to taste.

Ladle the venison into a large ovenproof dish, then carefully spoon on the creamy celeriac. Use a fork to encourage the mash to the edges of the dish and give it a little texture. Drizzle with a little olive oil, then pop the dish into the oven and bake for around 40 minutes, until golden and bubbling. Serve straight to the table with a mound of lemon-dressed greens.

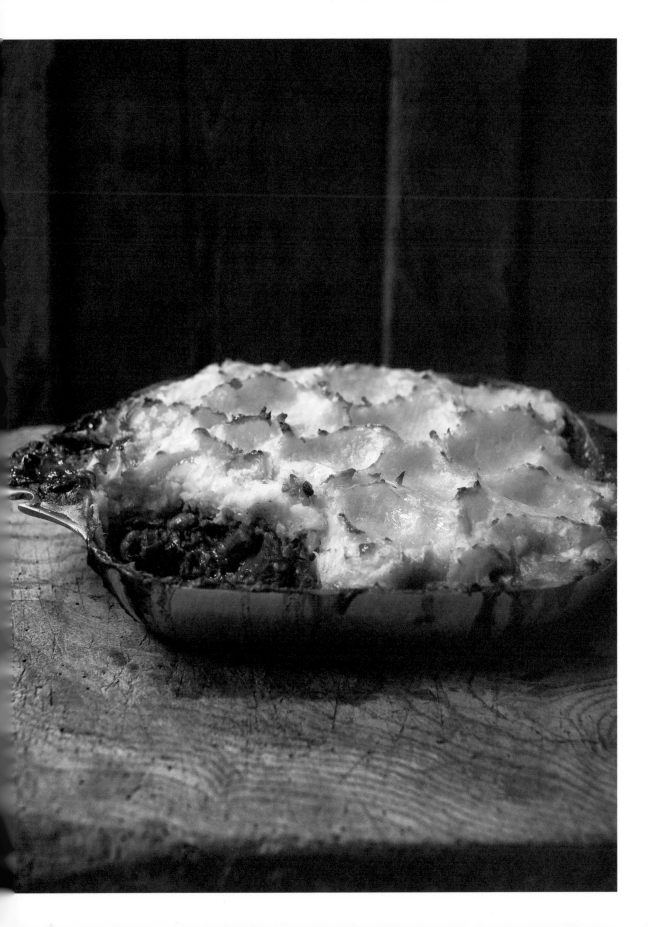

ROASTED GUINEA FOWL AND PUMPKIN PASTILLA

No trip to Morocco is complete without some form of pastilla. Traditionally filled with pigeon or even chicken, this delicious savoury and slightly sweet pie is a thing of beauty. The icing sugar finish may feel strange but don't skip it – it makes the dish.

SERVES 4–6

—

1 x 1–1.2kg guinea fowl

1 teaspoon ground cinnamon

½ teaspoon ground coriander

sea salt and freshly ground black
   pepper

olive oil

700g pumpkin or squash

3 red onions

½ teaspoon ground allspice

½ a bunch of coriander

½ a bunch of flat-leaf parsley

40g flaked almonds

60g butter

270g filo pastry

2 tablespoons icing sugar

250g Greek yoghurt

2 tablespoons harissa

Preheat your oven to 180°C/gas 4. Place the guinea fowl in a large roasting tray and sprinkle with ¼ teaspoon of ground cinnamon, the ground coriander, a good pinch of salt and pepper, and a drizzle of olive oil, and rub into the meat. Place in the oven and roast for 20 minutes.

Meanwhile peel the pumpkin or squash and chop into 2½–3cm pieces. Peel and trim the red onions and cut into 1cm wedges. When the guinea fowl has had 20 minutes in the oven, remove the tray and scatter the prepared veg around the bird. Sprinkle with ½ teaspoon of ground cinnamon and the allspice. Drizzle the veg with olive oil, toss it all together and return the tray to the oven for a further 45–50 minutes, until the meat is cooked through and the veg are soft and a little caramelised. Remove from the oven, but don't turn the oven off.

Leave the tray and meat to cool for 15 minutes, then shred the meat off the carcass and straight into the tray. Mash the pumpkin lightly with a potato masher, keeping some of it a little chunky but using the rest to bring together the meat and onions. Finely chop the coriander and parsley, stalks and all, and stir into the filling with two-thirds of the almonds.

Melt the butter in a small pan and use a pastry brush to brush the inside of an ovenproof frying pan or pie dish, around 26cm in diameter. Layer the filo into the pan, brushing with butter as you go and leaving plenty hanging over the sides so you have enough to cover the top. Fill the filo with the guinea fowl mixture, then gather the excess pastry over the top, covering the pie completely. Brush with a little more melted butter and sprinkle with the remaining almonds.

Place the pan in the bottom of the oven and bake for 35–40 minutes, until golden and crisp. Remove from the oven, and leave the pie in the pan for 5 minutes. Dust with the remaining cinnamon and icing sugar. Serve sliced into wedges, with the harissa rippled through the yoghurt on the side.

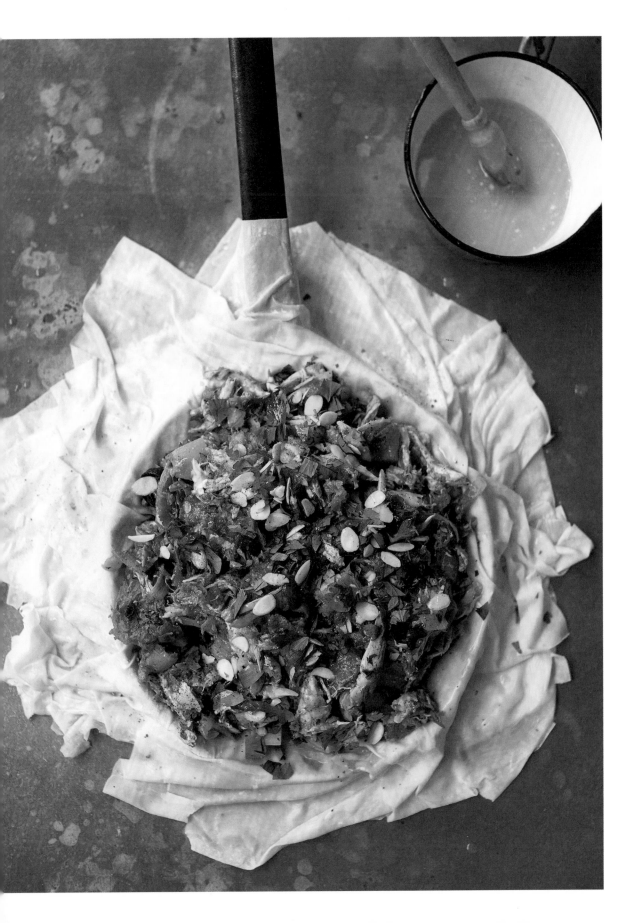

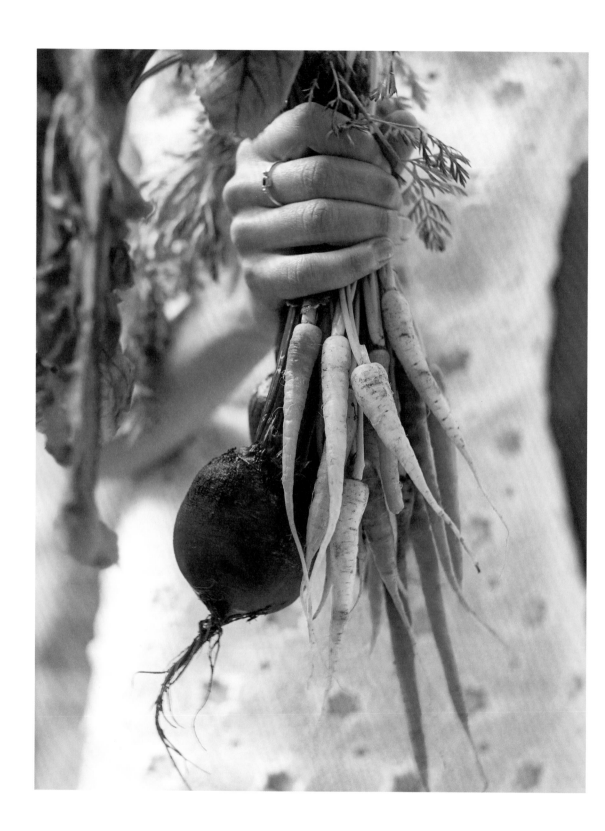

5

—

This chapter is a celebration of beautiful veg. These recipes make wonderful sides, but equally many of them are fantastic on their own, or as part of a group for a lighter meal. There isn't anything much better than a table filled with platters of beautifully and respectfully prepared vegetables and leaves.

GRIDDLED APRICOT, LETTUCE AND FETA

This is such a pretty little dish – the salty feta and sweet apricots work in perfect harmony. A simple summertime salad at its best.

SERVES 4
—

3 little gem lettuces

6 apricots, or 4 apricots and
  2 peaches

1 tablespoon runny honey

½ a bunch of mint

1 tablespoon white wine vinegar

3 tablespoons extra virgin olive oil

sea salt and freshly ground black
  pepper

125g feta

a good pinch of dried oregano

a punnet of micro cress *(optional)*

Preheat a griddle pan on a high heat. Trim the little gems, discard the outer leaves and cut into halves and then into quarters. Griddle the wedges, turning as you go so they are charred on all sides. When they're ready, take them off the griddle and put them on to a platter.

Cut the fruit in half and any large pieces in quarters, and remove the stones, then put them on the griddle, cut side down. You want to lightly caramelise the fruit, but be careful not to cook them for too long or they'll fall apart. As soon as they are ready, drizzle with a little honey and leave to one side while you make the dressing.

Pick the mint leaves and roughly chop. Put them into a bowl and whisk with the white wine vinegar, extra virgin olive oil and a good pinch of sea salt and freshly ground black pepper. Dot the griddled fruit around the little gem wedges on the platter . Drizzle with the mint dressing, and crumble over the feta. Finish with a scattering of dried oregano, snip over the micro cress if using, and serve straight away.

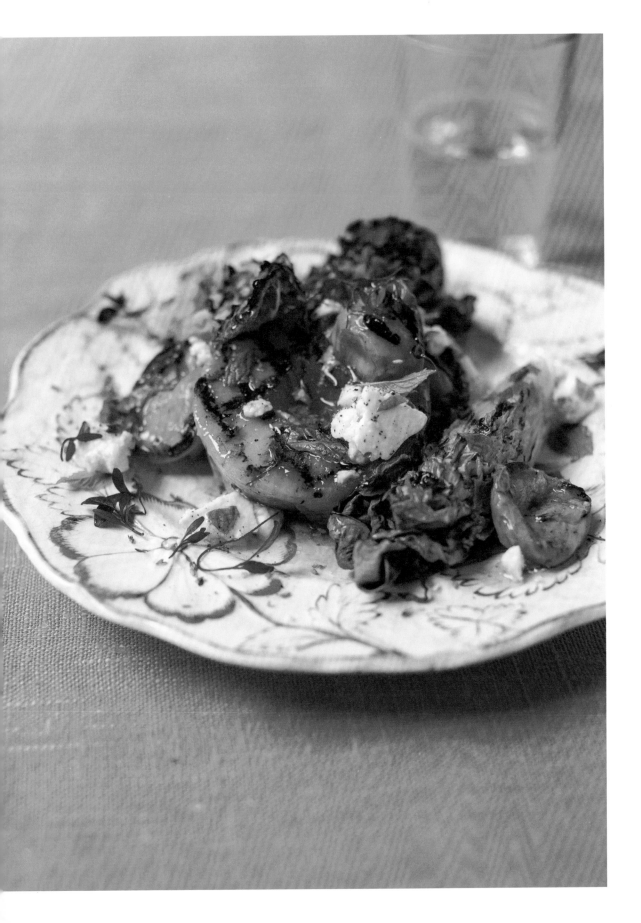

GARDEN SALAD WITH BUTTERMILK DRESSING AND CARAMELISED SEEDS

A simple green salad, with a creamy yet light mustardy dressing. The sweet and salty seeds are an absolute must.

SERVES 6
—

50g pumpkin seeds

1 tablespoon sesame seeds

50g sunflower seeds

100g caster sugar

sea salt and freshly ground black
    pepper

2 soft round lettuces

2 little gem lettuces

2 red chicory

1 teaspoon English mustard

zest and juice of 1 lemon

rapeseed oil

150ml buttermilk

a bunch of chives, finely chopped
    *(flowers too, if you can get
    them)*

Line a tray with greaseproof paper. Place a non-stick frying pan on a medium heat and toast all the seeds until lightly golden. Sprinkle in the sugar and a generous pinch of salt and gently caramelise until all the sugar has dissolved. Don't stir or it will form large crystals. Gently swirl the pan until you have a gorgeous golden caramel, then pour the mixture on to the prepared tray. Leave to one side to cool.

Cut off the lettuce leaves, wash and spin dry. Alternatively cut the lettuces and endives into large wedges, through the stem so that the wedges stay in one piece. Rinse, if needed, and dry with kitchen paper. Arrange them over a serving platter and leave to one side.

To make the dressing, spoon the mustard into a jam jar, season well and finely grate in the lemon zest. Squeeze in the lemon juice and add a couple of drizzles of rapeseed oil. Shake well until thoroughly mixed, then pour in the buttermilk and shake again.

In a mortar and pestle crush the caramelised seeds so you have a mixture of fine and chunky pieces. Finely chop the chives. Drizzle the buttermilk dressing over the salad, and scatter over the chives and the crushed seeds. Finish with any chive flowers, if you have them.

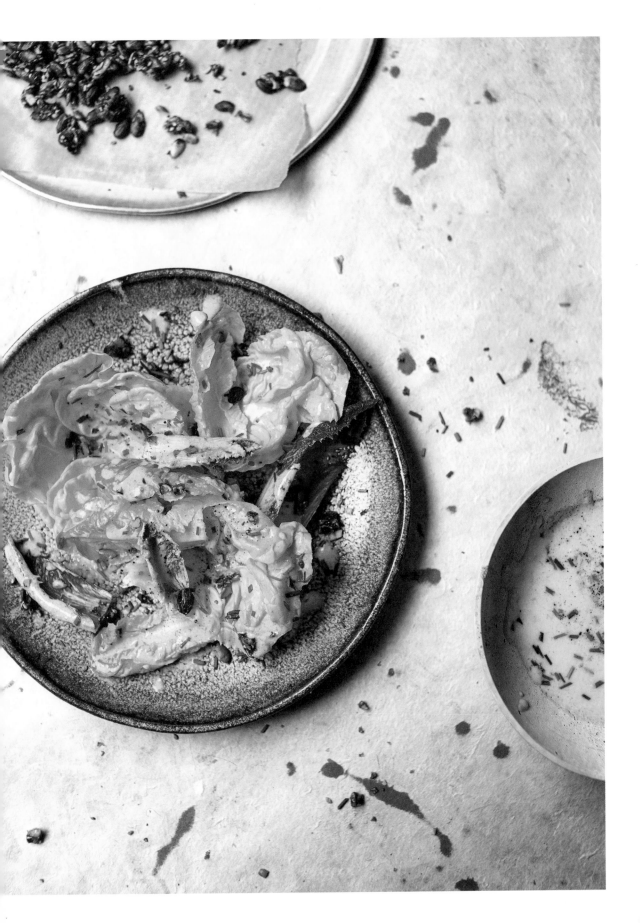

A VERY SPRINGTIME SALAD

This recipe does exactly what it says on the tin: delicious springtime ingredients, with little pops of creamy spiced labneh. Heaven.

SERVES 4, as a side or light lunch
—

1 teaspoon coriander seeds

1 teaspoon nigella seeds

2 teaspoons sesame seeds

1 lemon

1 teaspoon English mustard

extra virgin olive oil *(rapeseed or avocado oil work well too)*

sea salt and freshly ground black pepper

2 courgettes

4 spring onions

75g rocket

50g watercress

a handful of freshly podded peas

a handful of freshly podded broad beans, slipped out of their skins *(or just use more peas if you can't find them)*

a bunch of mixed soft herbs, such as parsley, mint, chervil, tarragon

150g labneh *(see page 240, or for a quicker alternative you can use a soft goat's cheese)*

Place a frying pan on a medium heat and scatter in the coriander, nigella and sesame seeds. Toast for a few minutes, until they're smelling great, then remove from the heat. Leave to cool, then coarsely grind in a mortar and pestle and leave to one side.

Make the dressing by whisking together the juice of the lemon, the mustard and 4 tablespoons of your oil. Season generously.

Trim the courgettes and spring onions. Finely slice the spring onions and place in a very large salad or mixing bowl. Using a potato peeler, slice the courgettes into long thin ribbons directly into the bowl. Wash and spin dry the rocket and watercress, and add to the bowl along with the podded peas and broad beans. Toss together gently.

Pick all the herb leaves and roughly chop together. Add most of them to the bowl, but reserve a couple of tablespoons and chop them finely. Add the ground seeds to the chopping board, with a generous pinch of salt, and mix with the herbs. Break the labneh into mouthful-size pieces (irregular is good! – they don't have to be perfect) and gently roll them in the spiced herb mixture. Dress the green salad with the lemon mustard dressing, scatter over the coated labneh, and serve.

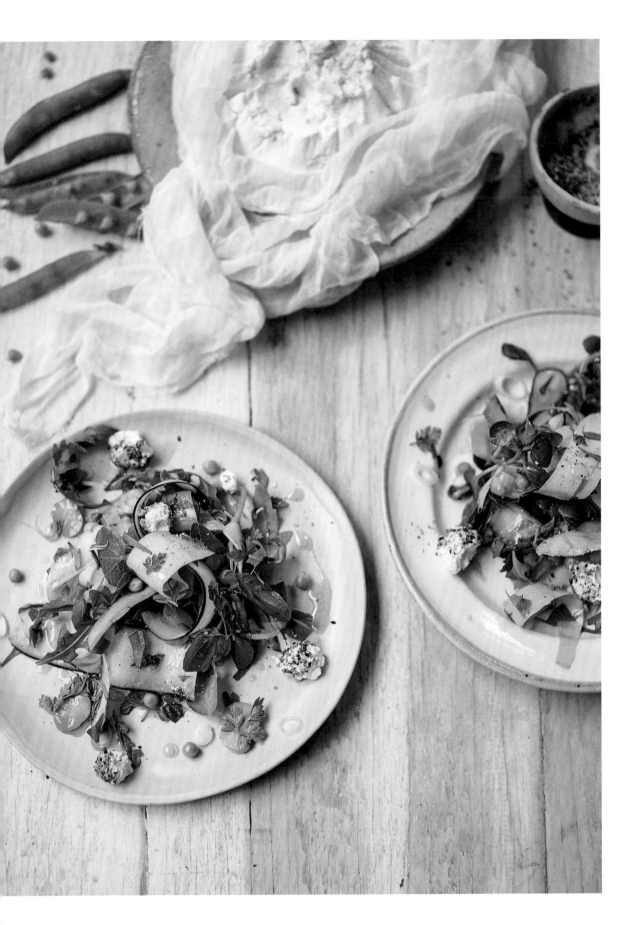

GRIDDLED RADICCHIO WITH HAZELNUT AND ROSEMARY

I absolutely adore this recipe – the contrast between the bitter leaves and the sweet dressing is heavenly. And if you've never tried griddling radicchio, I urge you to give it a go. It mellows the bitterness ever so slightly, and adds a lovely charred flavour to the salad.

SERVES 4-6

—

2 garlic cloves

40g hazelnuts

2 sprigs of rosemary

2 large or 3 medium radicchio

extra virgin olive oil

2 tablespoons dried cranberries

2 tablespoons runny honey

75ml balsamic vinegar

a handful of rocket leaves

100g good stale bread *(ciabatta or sourdough)*

sea salt and freshly ground black pepper

Place your griddle pan on a high heat and give it a few minutes to get screaming hot. Peel and finely slice the garlic. Roughly chop the hazelnuts. Pick the rosemary leaves and chop also. Cut the radicchio into large wedges, and when the pan is searing hot, pop the pieces on to char. Give them a few minutes on all sides, until you have good griddle marks, then place in a large serving bowl.

Pop a medium-size frying pan on a medium-low heat, pour in a glug of olive oil and add the garlic, hazelnuts, cranberries and rosemary leaves. Fry gently until the garlic turns a light golden colour, then add the honey and give it a minute to completely warm through. Pour the balsamic into the pan, stir it all together and turn the heat up. As soon as it starts to bubble, remove from the heat and leave the dressing to cool a little.

Wash the rocket and spin dry. Place the slightly cooled grilled radicchio on a chopping board and roughly chop it. Pop it back into the serving bowl. Chop the stale bread into mouthful-size pieces and add to the bowl too. Pour over the dressing, once it has cooled for 5 minutes, and toss everything together well. Season to taste, and finish by scattering over the rocket.

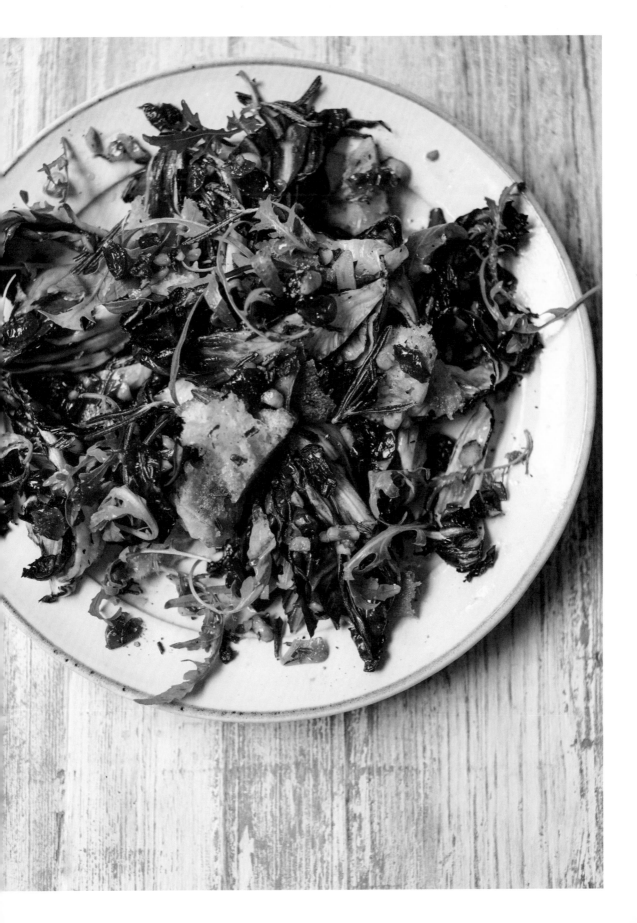

CHARRED BRASSICAS WITH TAHINI YOGHURT AND SUMAC

When roasted or barbecued, brassicas take on another dimension – meatier and more intense. Served here with a delicious rub and a tangy Greek yoghurt dressing – these are flavours that remind me of my summers in Cyprus. I could happily eat a whole bowl of this alone for my dinner.

SERVES 6, as a side

—

a pinch of saffron

½ teaspoon dried chilli flakes

1 heaped teaspoon dried oregano

½ tablespoon toasted sesame seeds *(a mixture of black and white if you can get both)*

sea salt and freshly ground black pepper

1kg brassicas *(I like to mix it up and use a head of broccoli and a head of romanesco cauliflower, when I can find them)*

olive oil

sea salt and freshly ground black pepper

250g Greek yoghurt

2 tablespoons tahini

1 lemon

½ a garlic clove

¼ teaspoon sumac

Preheat your oven to 200°/gas 6.

Place the saffron in a small bowl or teacup and cover with 2 tablespoons of just-boiled water. Give it a stir, then leave to one side.

In a mortar and pestle bash together the chilli flakes, oregano, sesame seeds and 1 teaspoon of sea salt until you have a finer-textured salt.

Slice your veg up into a mixture of florets and slices, including the stalks, so that they are evenly sized, and spread them over a couple of roasting trays. Evenly drizzle with olive oil and sprinkle over all the flavoured salt. Toss everything together, then spread out into one layer. Pop into the oven for 25–30 minutes, and roast until the veg are just cooked through but lovely and charred at the edges.

While the brassicas are in the oven, make the yoghurt dressing. Spoon the yoghurt and tahini into a mixing bowl and squeeze in the lemon juice; mix until smooth. Peel and finely grate in the garlic and season well. The saffron water should now be cool, and a vibrant gold colour. Pour the liquid – saffron threads and all – into the yoghurt, and stir it through.

Spread the yoghurt on your serving platter, and when the veg are ready arrange them on top. Finish by sprinkling over the sumac, and serve. Delicious served at room temperature too, making it a great get-ahead side dish.

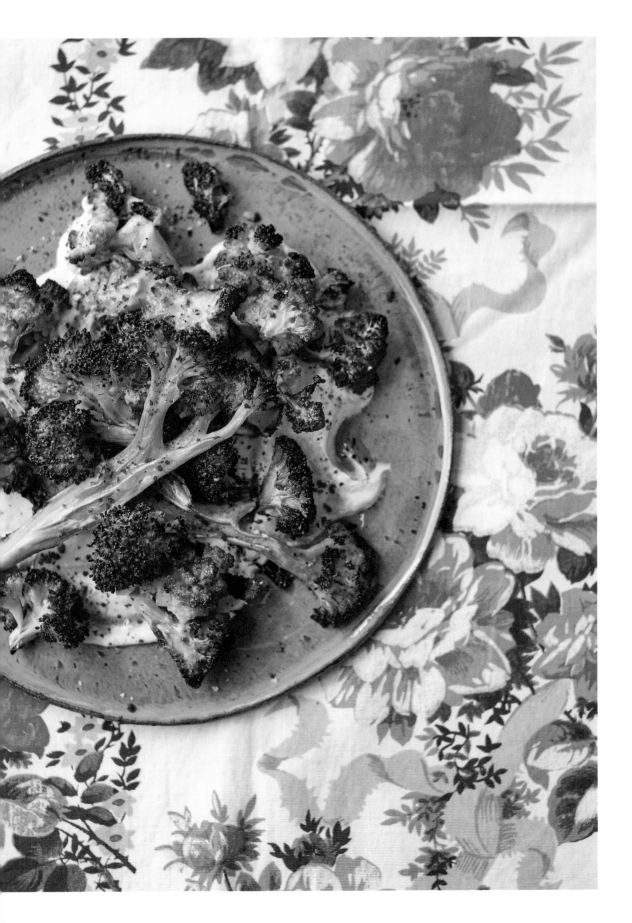

KHICHDI

I adore this recipe. It's a traditional Indian dish which is nourishing both to make and to eat - it's filled with goodness and follows a lot of the Ayurvedic principles. I think it is perfect as a side for a Indian meal or just on its own, in a bowl, with a spoon. Make a batch on a Sunday and it'll keep you going for a few days.

SERVES 6

—

150g split mung beans

3 garlic cloves

2 onions

1 green chilli

a 2cm piece of ginger

3 tablespoons ghee

½ tablespoon cumin seeds

250g basmati rice (*I like to use white and brown*)

sea salt and freshly ground black pepper

15 curry leaves

1 teaspoon black mustard seeds

1 teaspoon ground turmeric

1 small cinnamon stick

200g kale or spinach

Wash the mung beans in a sieve under running water. Peel and finely slice the garlic, and peel and finely chop the onions. Halve, deseed and finely slice the chilli. Peel the ginger and keep to one side.

Heat a little of the ghee in a large saucepan over a medium heat and add the cumin seeds. Once they start to turn golden and smell wonderful, add the rice and mung beans to the pan. Season well with salt and pepper and add 1.75 litres of water. Bring to the boil, then reduce to a simmer and cover with a lid. Leave to cook on a low heat for 40 minutes, adding more water if it gets a little dry.

While the rice and mung beans are cooking, you can temper the rest of the spices. To do this, heat the rest of the ghee in a frying pan over a medium heat and add the garlic. Fry for a minute and once the garlic has turned lightly golden, add the onions, chilli and curry leaves, and finely grate in the ginger. Turn the heat down a little and sauté for 5–10 minutes, until the onions have softened but not coloured. Turn the heat up a little and add the mustard seeds, turmeric and cinnamon stick. Fry for 2 more minutes.

Wash the greens thoroughly and remove any tough stalks, then roughly chop and add to the pan along with the sautéed spiced onions and a splash of water, if needed. You want a creamy texture, so add up to 200ml of water if it feels too thick. Cook for a further 15–20 minutes, then season to taste. Perfect with warm chapatis and a feast of other Indian dishes.

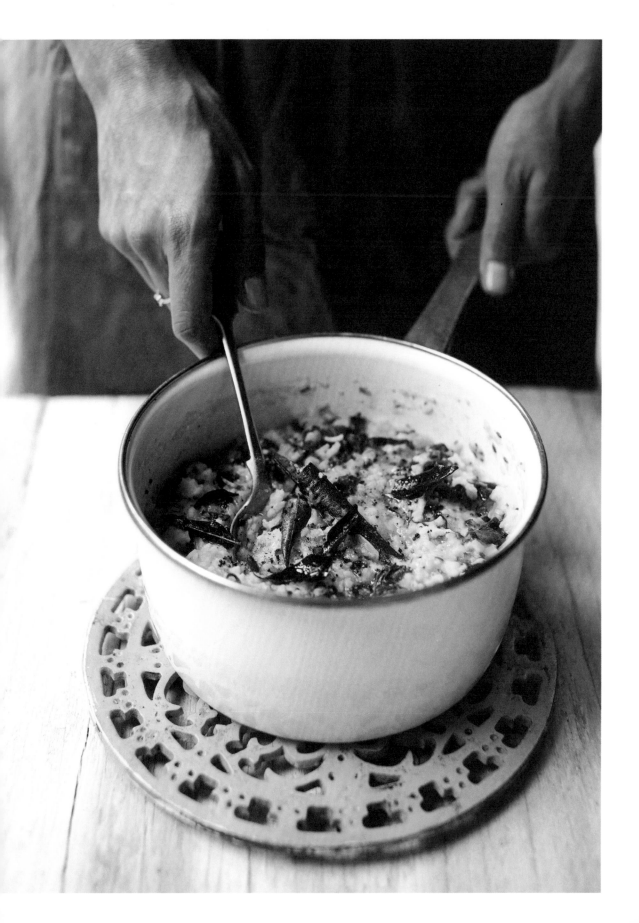

INDULGENT POLENTA WITH ROASTED GARLIC BUTTER

Done well, polenta has to be one of the most comforting foods of all time; done badly, it's a stodgy mess. Don't let this put you off, though! It isn't hard to do at all, you just need a little time, patience and the ability to turn a blind eye to the butter and salt content. This would be perfect with the cinnamon-braised lamb shanks on page 160, or by itself in a bowl with a pile of greens for good measure.

NB This recipe makes more garlic butter than you need for the polenta, as it's easier to roast a whole bulb of garlic at a time. There are different ways to roast a bulb of garlic, but I just pop a bulb in the oven when something else is already cooking, and leave it to caramelise. Just store the rest in the fridge and use it another day, with potatoes, chicken, veg – it's delicious!

SERVES 4

—

a whole bulb of garlic

extra virgin olive oil

a bunch of basil

150g butter

sea salt and freshly ground black pepper

250ml milk

150g coarse polenta *(not the quick-cook stuff)*

50g pecorino

Preheat your oven to 180°C/gas 4. Peel away some of the papery layers from the garlic bulb and drizzle with oil. Place the bulb in a small ovenproof dish and pop into the oven for 1hr 15 minutes, until it is soft, golden and starting to look sticky. Leave to one side to cool a little before making the butter.

Chop the basil, stalks and all. Cut 125g of butter into chunks and pop into a food processor with the basil and a good pinch of seasoning. Squeeze the garlic cloves out of their skins and into the blender. Blitz until you have a vibrant green butter. Spoon on to a sheet of greaseproof paper, roll into a log and store in the fridge until needed.

To make the polenta, pour the milk into a large heavy-based pan along with 750ml of water and just under a teaspoon of sea salt. Gently bring to the boil, then slowly and steadily pour the polenta into the pan in a thin stream, whisking all the time so it thickens as you go. Keep whisking for a couple of minutes over a high heat. Turn the heat down to the lowest setting and cook the polenta for around 40 minutes, until it starts to come away from the pan, stirring every 5 minutes to stop it sticking.

When it's ready, finely grate in the pecorino, stir in the remaining 25g of butter, season to taste and stir well.

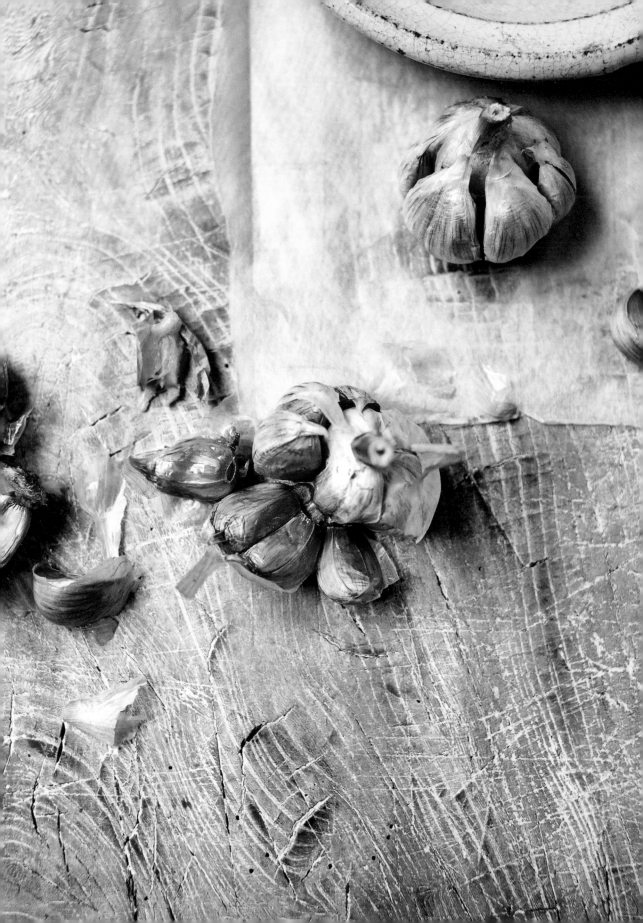

WHOLE ROASTED MISO AUBERGINE

I've met quite a few people who don't love aubergine, and I can honestly say most of the time it's because of the way it's cooked. That rubbery, dry, slightly squeaky texture is pretty off-putting, but that's purely because it hasn't been cooked for long enough. Aubergines are a beautiful thing, and when given the right care they are stunning. Take this recipe, for example – I treat the aubergines like a piece of meat, slashing them, marinating them and slow-roasting them whole. The result is a deliciously creamy and fragrant dish that takes little effort to make. The other bonus is that you don't use much oil, as you cook the aubergines whole, so it's light too.

SERVES 4
—

a 3cm piece of ginger

4 garlic cloves

2 small green chillies

2 aubergines

sea salt and freshly ground black pepper

groundnut oil

200g vine cherry tomatoes

4 spring onions

½ a bunch of coriander

1 lime

1 tablespoon tamarind paste

½ tablespoon honey

3 tablespoons white sweet miso

Preheat your oven to 180°C/gas 4.

Peel the ginger and garlic, and finely slice the chillies. Pierce the aubergines all over with a paring knife, as if you were making incisions into a piece of meat. Grate the ginger into a large mortar and pestle, and bash together with the garlic, chillies and a good pinch of salt until you have a thick paste. Mix in just enough oil to make it spoonable, place the aubergines in a large roasting tray, then spoon the mixture over the aubergines and massage it into the incisions, really getting the flavours inside. Dot the cherry tomatoes around, and pop into the oven for 40 minutes, turning the aubergines a couple of times.

While the aubergines are cooking, trim and finely slice the spring onions and roughly chop the coriander, stalks and all. Put into a bowl, squeeze over the lime juice to coat and mix all together. Leave to one side.

Mix together the tamarind, honey and miso and add enough water to make a thick glaze. Remove the roasting tray from the oven after 40 minutes, turn the oven up to 200°C/gas 6, and drizzle the miso glaze over the aubergines. Pop back into the oven for a further 20 minutes, to caramelise, then remove and leave to cool a little.

Working carefully, remove the stalks from the aubergines and discard them, then roughly chop the flesh in the tray into coarse chunks. Stir in the dressed spring onions and coriander and serve right away.

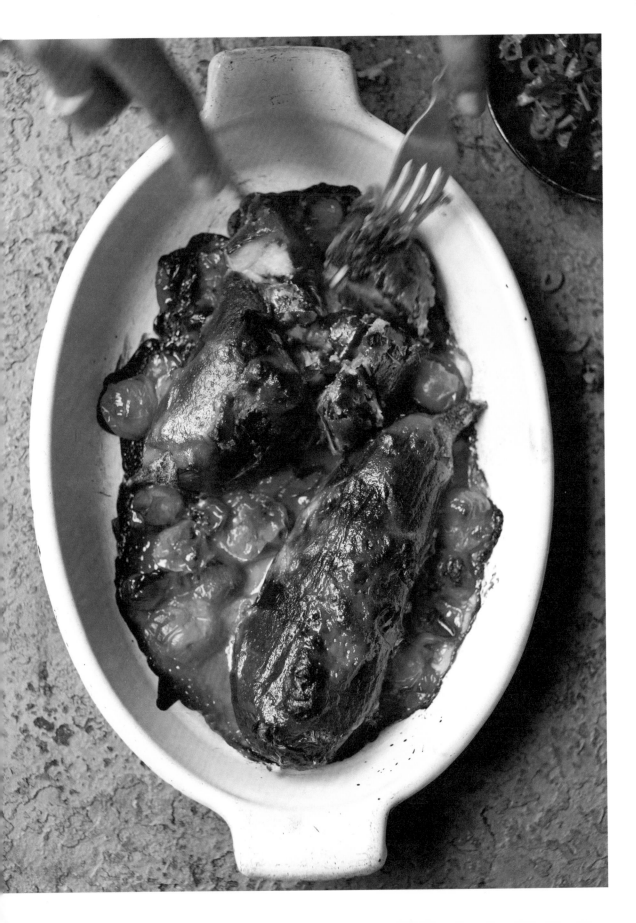

TOMATO, BREAD AND ROASTED RICOTTA SALAD

During the summer months I will frequently make this for myself for lunch. It is loosely based on the famous Italian 'panzanella', which is summer in a bowl – sweet, light and fresh. However, I don't rely on stale bread, as bread doesn't seem to last long enough in our house to go stale. Instead I roast it, and I also like to introduce a little creaminess into the salad for which ricotta is perfect. You don't have to roast it, straight up works well too – roasting just gives the cheese an interesting and robust texture.

SERVES 4 as a main, or 6-8 as a side

—

200g good-quality ricotta

extra virgin olive oil

½ teaspoon dried oregano

sea salt and freshly ground black pepper

a loaf of ciabatta *(about 275g)*

1 bunch of basil

1 small garlic clove

2 tablespoons red wine vinegar

1kg ripe vine tomatoes, a mix of colour and sizes if possible

1 green chilli

Preheat your oven to 180°/gas 4.

Put the ricotta into a small roasting tray or dish, drizzle with a good glug of olive oil, and sprinkle over the oregano. Season well, then pop into the oven for 30 minutes, until golden on the outside. When there are 10 minutes left to go, tear the ciabatta into mouthful-size pieces and scatter into a roasting tray. Drizzle with oil, season well and pop into the oven to crisp up for 10 minutes. When the ricotta and bread are both ready, remove from the oven and leave to one side to cool.

Meanwhile make the dressing. Roughly chop the basil and peel the garlic, then place both in a blender along with the red wine vinegar. Season, and pour in around 4 tablespoons of extra virgin olive oil. Blitz until you have a smooth green dressing, adding a little more oil if it is too thick.

Slice and erratically chop the tomatoes and place in a large bowl – I like to have a mixture of shapes and sizes. Add the toasted ciabatta and the basil dressing, mix everything together, and leave for 10 minutes to soften. When the salad is ready, transfer it to a serving platter and crumble over the roasted ricotta. Halve and deseed the chilli, slice as finely as you can, scatter over the top, along with any leftover basil leaves, and serve.

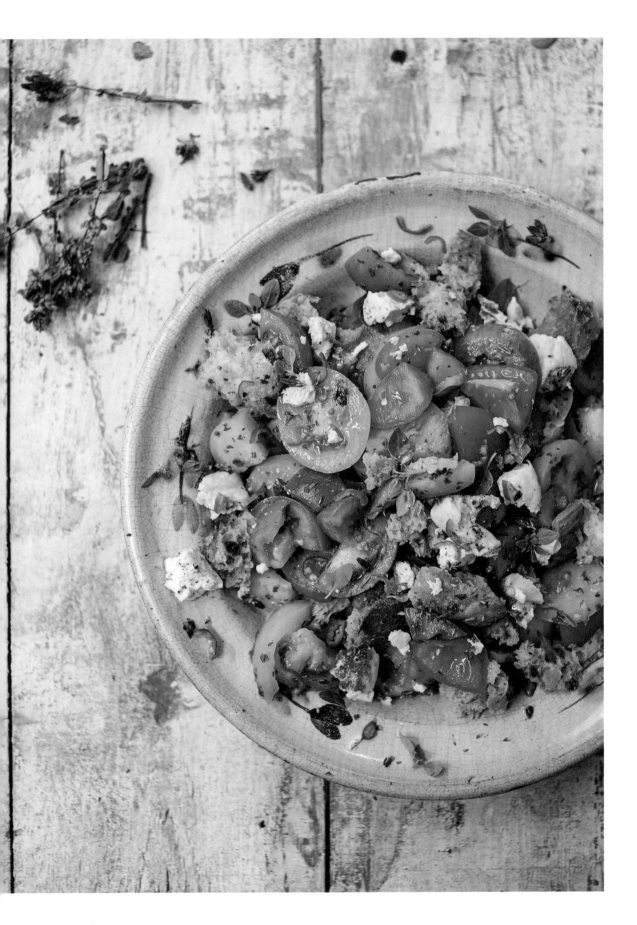

HONEYMOON CORN ON THE COB

We became addicted to spiced corn on the cob while on our honeymoon in Indonesia. You'll find a flurry of corn sellers pushing their carts up and down the beaches in the late afternoon, just in time for sundowners and snacks, each with their own spiced butter to finish. Here I have tried to recreate my favourite; the combination of salty, sweet and spicy is heavenly. Perfect for a party, barbecue, or even just an afternoon snack. Any unused butter can be stored in the fridge for another day.

SERVES 8

—

a 2cm piece of ginger

2 garlic cloves

2 limes

sea salt

1 red chilli

1 stick of lemongrass

1 heaped tablespoon light soft
brown sugar

150g unsalted butter

8 corn on the cob, in their husks if
possible

Peel and roughly chop the ginger and garlic and put into a mortar and pestle. Finely grate in the lime zest, add a generous pinch of sea salt and bash until you have a smooth paste. Halve the chilli, remove the seeds and chop; add to the mortar and bash it a bit more to work it in. Trim the lemongrass and remove the outer layers, then add to the paste. Crush it so it breaks up a little, then mix in the brown sugar and a little more salt.

Cut the butter into chunks and pop into a small saucepan. Spoon in the spice paste and place the pan on a low heat. Very gently melt the butter, stirring occasionally. Once it has completely melted, keep it on a low heat for a further 5 minutes, to make sure all the flavours infuse as much as possible. Remove the pan from the heat and leave to one side to cool completely. Once cool, pour it into a small bowl and pop it into the fridge until needed. You can make this hours, even days, in advance.

If you are using corn cobs in their husks, be sure to soak them in plenty of water for at least an hour before you want to grill them, otherwise the husks will burn. Put your griddle on to a high heat. If you are grilling the corn cobs in their husks, you'll need to cook them for around 20 minutes; peeled, they'll only need around 15 minutes. Turn the cobs occasionally, and when they are ready peel back the husks (or not, if already peeled) and brush on the butter. Griddle for a further few minutes on each side, brushing as you go to build up a good coat of flavour. Place on a board or platter, brushing with one final layer of butter. Cut the limes into wedges, and serve alongside.

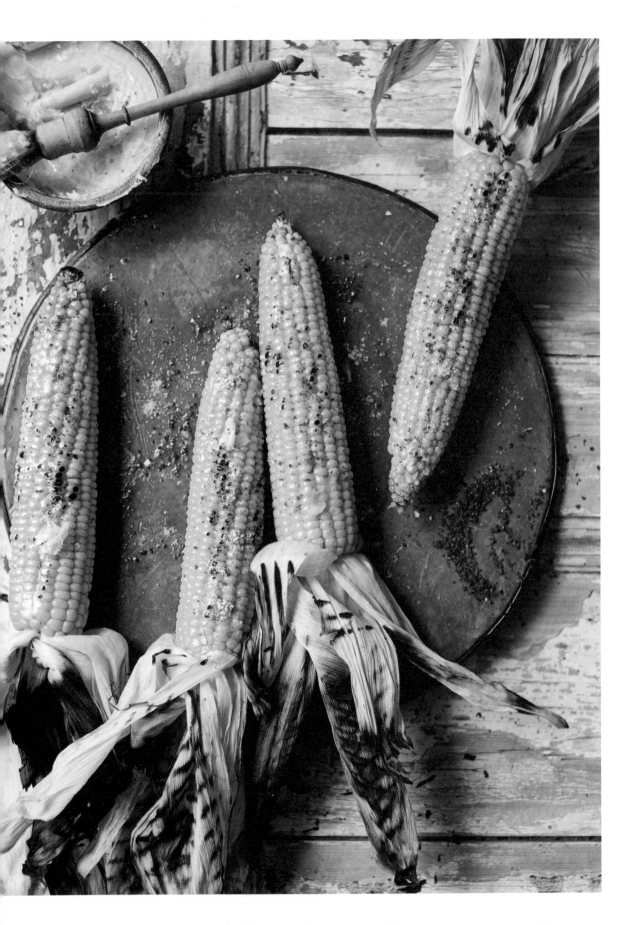

APPLE, PEAR AND TARRAGON SLAW

This shredded salad is crisp and refreshing, making it the perfect accompaniment to heartier meals (I love it on the side of the leftover mac 'n' cheese on page 148).

SERVES 6
—

2 English apples, such as Cox's or Braeburn

2 small or 1 large firm pear

½ a lemon

1 small onion

a bunch of tarragon

3 tablespoons cider vinegar

1 teaspoon Dijon mustard

extra virgin olive oil

sea salt and freshly ground black pepper

50g salad leaves such as watercress, baby beet, rocket

a punnet of salad cress

Trim the apples and pears, then, using a mandolin, or the slicing attachment on a food processor, slice them as finely as possible. Put them into a large bowl and squeeze over the juice of the lemon half to stop them browning. Peel and halve the onion and finely slice also, then add to the bowl. Toss everything together and leave to one side.

Pick the tarragon leaves and pop them into a blender with the cider vinegar, mustard and 4 tablespoons of extra virgin olive oil. Season well, then blitz it all together until you have a vibrant green dressing. If need be, loosen with a little more oil, then pour over the fruit. Mix it all together with your hands, making sure everything is well dressed. Wash and spin dry the watercress and add it to the bowl. Snip in the salad cress, mix it together one last time and serve straight away.

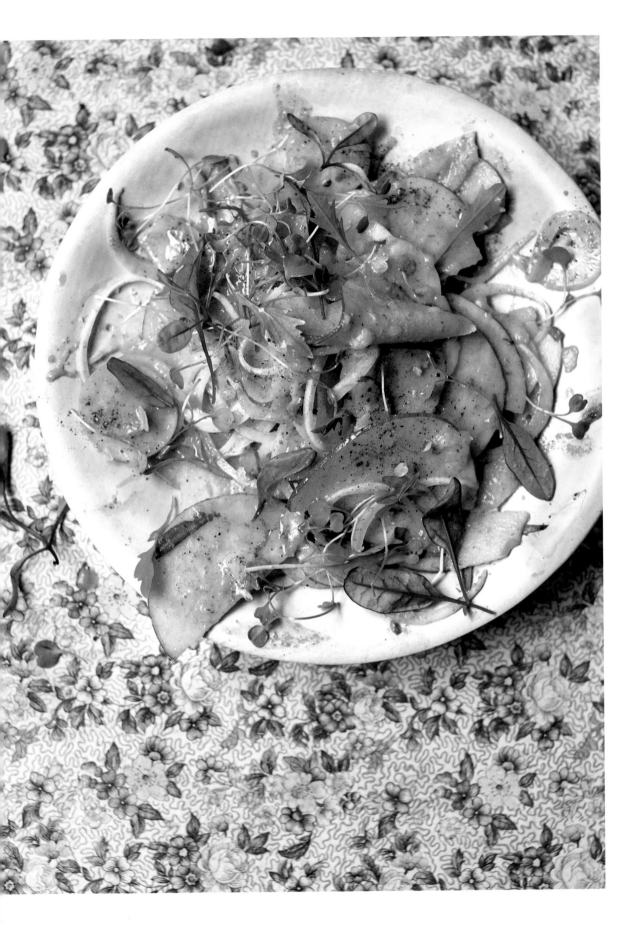

STICKY HARISSA CARROTS AND BEETS WITH DATES

If I'm making this, I'll make double, just so there are plenty of leftovers for the next day. It's such a simple and flavoursome dish, and works wonderfully as part of a sit-down meal, buffet and even in your lunchbox. I could eat this till the cows come home.

SERVES 6
—

900g carrots and golden beetroots *(you can use other beetroots if you can't find golden, or even use just carrots)*

2 tablespoons harissa *(I love rose harissa)*

1 orange or 2 clementines

olive oil

sea salt and freshly ground black pepper

1 heaped tablespoon honey

2 tablespoons mixed seeds, such as pumpkin, sesame and sunflower

a bunch of flat-leaf parsley

75g medjool dates

a splash of red wine vinegar

Preheat the oven to 200°C/gas 6. Bring a large pan of salted water to the boil.

Peel and trim the carrots and beetroots. Chop into mouthful-size chunks, around 3–4cm, and pop them into the pan of boiling water. Parboil for 5 minutes, then drain and leave to steam dry for a minute. Scatter the veg into a large roasting tray and spoon over the harissa. Halve the orange or clementines and squeeze over the juice. Drizzle with a good glug of olive oil, season well and toss everything together until evenly coated. Place the tray in the oven for 30 minutes, giving it a shake halfway through. After half an hour, drizzle the veg evenly with the honey, then return to the oven for a further 10–15 minutes, until sticky and gnarly.

If your seeds are untoasted, scatter them on a baking tray and pop them into the oven for the last 4–5 minutes, until lightly toasted and golden.

Leave the veg and seeds to one side for about 10 minutes to cool. Pick and chop the parsley leaves. Remove the stones from the dates and finely chop. When the veg and seeds have cooled a little, toss the parsley, chopped dates and seeds into the veg along with a tablespoon of red wine vinegar. Taste and tweak the seasoning, adding more vinegar if needed, then spoon on to a platter or into a large bowl and serve.

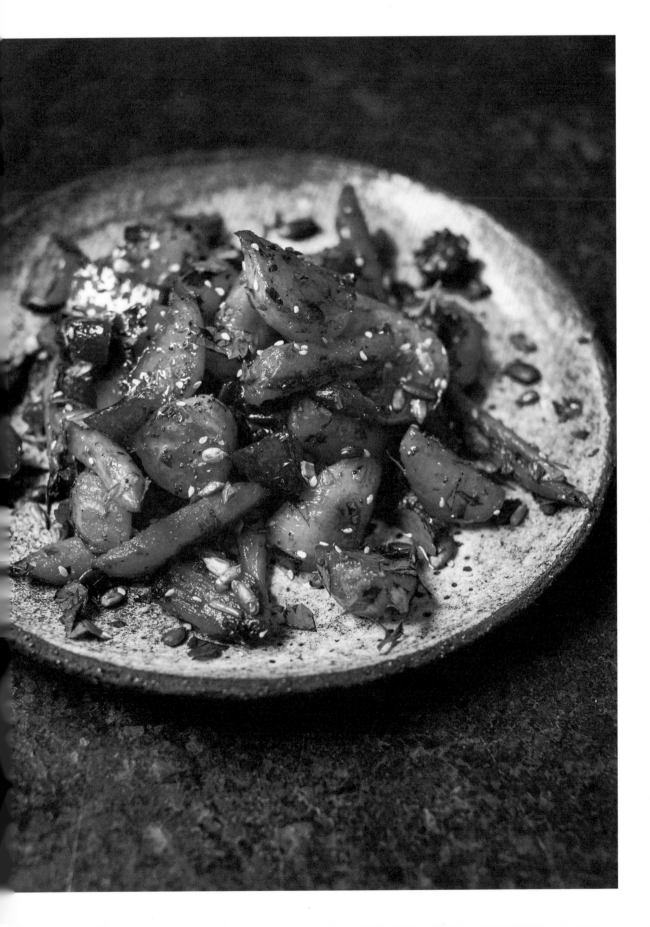

KILLER DRESSED ROAST POTATOES

When I was growing up (and even now occasionally), my yiayias were both renowned for their amazing roast potatoes. It wasn't until recently that I realised the reason they were so good was that they'd confit them in a pan of oil on the hob! Delicious, but heart-attack worthy. We've reined in the confited veg now and I much prefer the chuffing and roasting method. This is my favourite way of serving my roast spuds, crisp and hit with delicious flavour at the last minute.

SERVES 6–8
—

1.5kg Maris Piper potatoes

sea salt and freshly ground black
  pepper

olive oil

¼ teaspoon good dried oregano

1 garlic clove

1 lemon

½ a bunch of parsley

½ a red chilli

Preheat your oven to 190°C/gas 5.

Peel the potatoes, leave the small ones whole and cut any larger ones so that they are all the same size. Place them in a large saucepan with a generous pinch of salt, cover with cold water and place on a high heat. Bring the water to the boil, then cook the potatoes for 10 minutes, so that they are almost cooked through. Drain them in the colander and leave them to steam dry for a few minutes.

Make sure the saucepan you cooked the potatoes in is completely dry, then transfer them back to the pan. Cover with the lid and shake the pan to really chuff them up. The outside of all the spuds should look broken down and fluffy.

Transfer the chuffed potatoes to a large roasting tray, so they sit in one layer, and drizzle with a good glug of olive oil. Season generously, sprinkle over the oregano and toss them all together. Place the tray in the oven and roast the potatoes for 1 hour and 20 minutes, scraping them and turning them once or twice during cooking.

When the potatoes are almost ready, make your dressing. Peel the garlic and finely grate on to a chopping board. Finely grate over the lemon zest and pick all the parsley leaves. Deseed and finely chop the chilli, then run your knife through everything together, chopping it all up so it is really fine. Squeeze over half the lemon juice and mix together well.

When the potatoes are ready and golden all over, spoon over the chopped herb dressing and toss through evenly. Serve straight away.

GREEN CHILLI GREENS WITH CASHEWS

The humble cabbage often gets overlooked nowadays in favour of its trendier neighbours – kale, chard and spinach. But they are all wonderful and will often react in a similar way. Cooking them the way I do here keeps them fresh and nutritious – you shouldn't end up with soggy overcooked greens. It also works beautifully with shredded sprouts – just cook them for a little less time. I love it as an accompaniment to curries and spicy foods, but it also makes a great alternative side to a Sunday roast dinner or pie.

SERVES 6

—

35g cashew nuts

450g green cabbage *(pointed or spring cabbage – you could also use Brussels sprouts)*

a 2cm piece of ginger

2 garlic cloves

sea salt and freshly ground black pepper

2 shallots

1–2 green chillies, *depending on how spicy you like your food*

groundnut oil or vegetable oil

½ tablespoon cumin seeds

1 teaspoon black mustard seeds

½ teaspoon turmeric

1 teaspoon ground coriander

½ a lemon

Preheat your oven to 180°C/gas 4. Scatter the cashew nuts on a small tray and roast in the oven for 8–10 minutes, until golden. Remove and leave to cool.

Trim the cabbage and discard any not so great outer leaves. Shred the cabbage as finely as you can. If using Brussels sprouts, trim the ends and shred the sprouts in a food processor on a slicing attachment, or very carefully by hand. Peel the ginger and garlic and roughly chop. Place them in a mortar and pestle with a good pinch of salt, and bash them until you have a paste. Peel the shallots and finely slice. Halve, deseed and finely slice the chillies.

Place a large frying pan on a medium-low heat and add a good drizzle of oil. Add the cumin seeds and mustard seeds and fry for a minute, so they start to pop. Add the sliced shallots and chillies to the pan. Spoon in the garlic and ginger paste, turmeric and ground coriander and sauté for 10 minutes, until softened but not coloured. Stir in the shredded cabbage, turn the heat up a little, and fry for 6–8 minutes, until softened. If it starts to catch, add a splash of water to the pan. If the cabbage is not quite done, leave it for a couple more minutes. Cook away any liquid left in the pan and squeeze in the juice from the lemon half.

While the cabbage is cooking finely chop the cashew nuts. When the cabbage is ready, stir in the nuts and serve straight away.

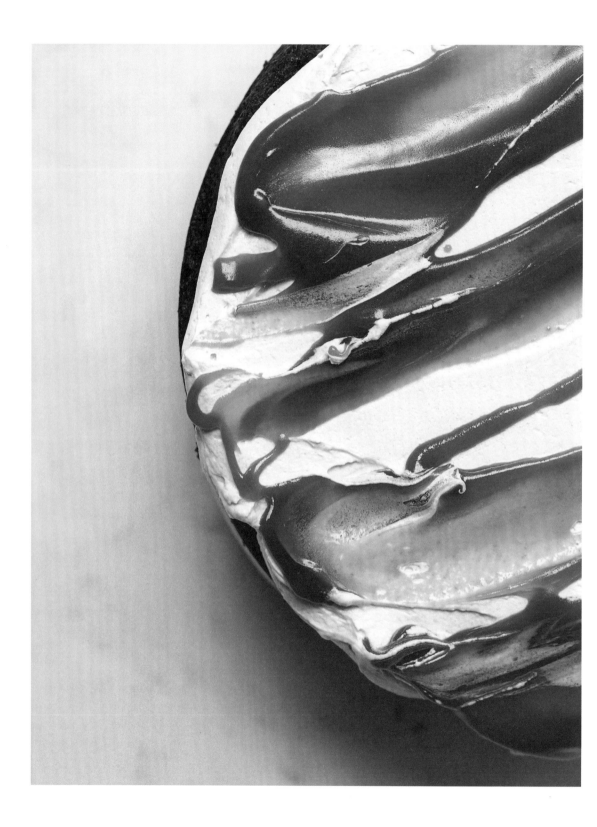

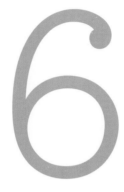

6

BAKE YOURSELF BETTER

—

For me baking is the ultimate form of kitchen therapy. I love every part of the baking process – the weighing out, the precision, the beating and folding, I even love the mess! Baking is truly something to lose yourself in. It's also food that needs to be shared, which is surely one of life's greatest simple pleasures: making something and sharing it with another. Also, turn up at someone's door with a home-baked item and you are guaranteed a smile. It's a beautiful thing. In this chapter you'll find some new recipes, some classics and some blowout showstopper pieces to really sink your teeth (and time) into.

ALMOND, OAT AND RAISIN COOKIES

If you make these cookies and do not eat at least a spoonful of the mixture before baking them, you have my full respect (or you're telling porkies). I've yet to make them and not devour the unbaked mix. This is my ultimate cookie – warming, familiar, moreish, chewy, comforting. I want these with a big mug of tea and a blanket while watching something on the TV that I've seen a million times before. They're the equivalent of a duvet day, but in cookie form.

MAKES AROUND 20

—

175g rolled oats

150g wholemeal or plain flour

a good pinch of sea salt

1 teaspoon ground cinnamon

1 teaspoon baking powder

125g butter, at room temperature

75g almond butter *(any nut butter will do – peanut is amazing also)*

325g soft light brown sugar

2 large eggs

100g raisins

Preheat the oven to 180°C/gas 4.

Blitz 100g of the oats in a food processor until finely ground. Add the flour, salt, ground cinnamon and baking powder and pulse to mix it all together. If you don't have a food processor, don't worry about it – the cookies are still delicious without the oats being blitzed.

Place the butter and almond butter in the bowl of a free-standing mixer and beat together for a minute till smooth. (Alternatively use a mixing bowl and an electric hand whisk.) Add the sugar and beat for a further 2–3 minutes, until pale and creamy. Beat in the eggs, then with a metal spoon fold in the dry mixture, the additional 75g of oats and the raisins.

Line a couple of baking sheets with greaseproof paper and spoon on tablespoonfuls of the mixture, a little larger than the size of a golfball – making sure you leave at least 2–3cm between them. Bake for 10–11 minutes, until starting to turn golden but still a little soft. Leave the cookies on the baking sheets for 5 minutes, then transfer to a rack to cool completely.

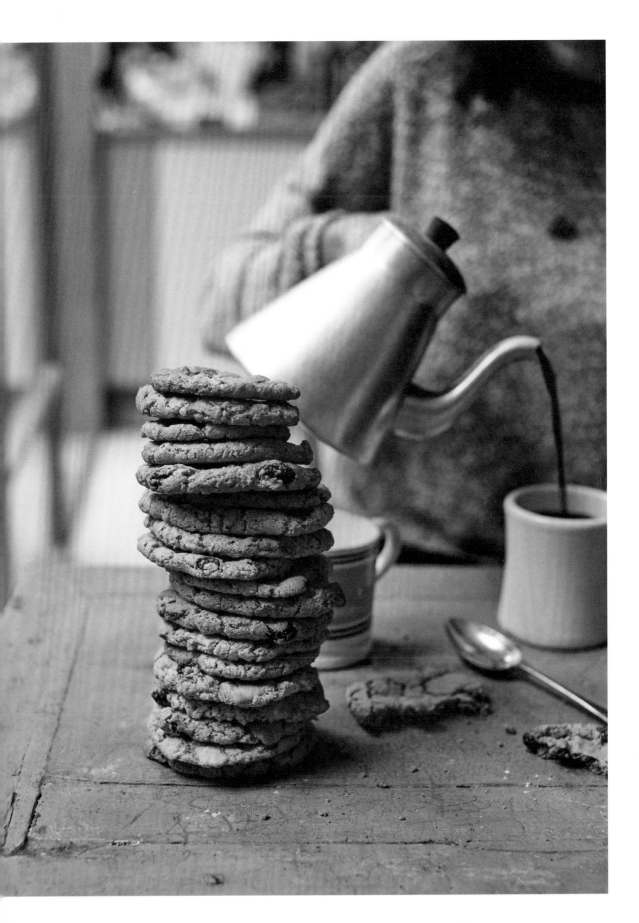

AN INSANELY GOOD BLONDIE

If you've got this far into the book you'll realise that I don't use coconut oil in any of my recipes. That's not because I don't like it – on the contrary, I think coconut oil can be delicious. But this wave of using it for everything isn't my cup of tea. Working alongside a team of nutritionists has taught me that it is higher in saturated fat than lard, and the so-called health benefits just don't outweigh that fact for me (if I'm frying an egg it'll be in olive oil – heck, if I fry anything, eight times out of ten it'll be olive oil). However, this is one recipe where I do use it. This started as a quest to create an incredible blondie, something moreish and standout. Brownies, blondies, cakes by default are not healthy items, and the addition of coconut oil really does create a great flavour. So please let me just clarify: I am not claiming in any way that these are healthy or good for you, they just taste delicious and are calming to make, and I am totally OK with that.

MAKES 20 PIECES

—

2 teaspoons baking powder

½ heaped teaspoon sea salt

250g plain flour

180g coconut oil or unsalted butter, or a mixture of both

300g soft light brown sugar

2 large eggs, beaten

1½ teaspoons vanilla extract

125g good-quality dark, milk or white chocolate, or a mix of chocolates

Preheat your oven to 180°C/gas 4. Grease a 20cm square cake tin and line with greaseproof paper. Whisk the baking powder, sea salt and plain flour in a bowl and leave to one side. Melt the coconut oil (and/or butter) in a medium pan, over a low heat. Add the sugar, breaking up any hard clumps, and dissolve slowly into the coconut oil. As soon as you have a golden caramel, remove the pan from the heat and pour into a large mixing bowl. (Don't worry if the sugar is a little grainy, it will come back again once you add the remaining ingredients.)

Leave to one side for 15 minutes, then whisk in the eggs and vanilla extract. Fold in the flour mixture with a large metal spoon, until everything is just mixed together – try not to over-beat it. Chop the chocolate into chunks and stir it in, then spoon the blondie mixture into the prepared tin. Smooth out into one even layer and pop into the oven for 30 minutes – until it is cooked, has a lovely crust but is still just a little soft.

Leave to cool in the tin for 10 minutes, then quickly and efficiently transfer to a cooling rack. Leave the blondies to cool for another 10 minutes, then cut into 20 pieces. Leave on the rack till completely cool, then store in a cake tin or Tupperware box for up to 3–4 days – if they make it that long. (Although weirdly I do think these taste better the next day...) Heavenly.

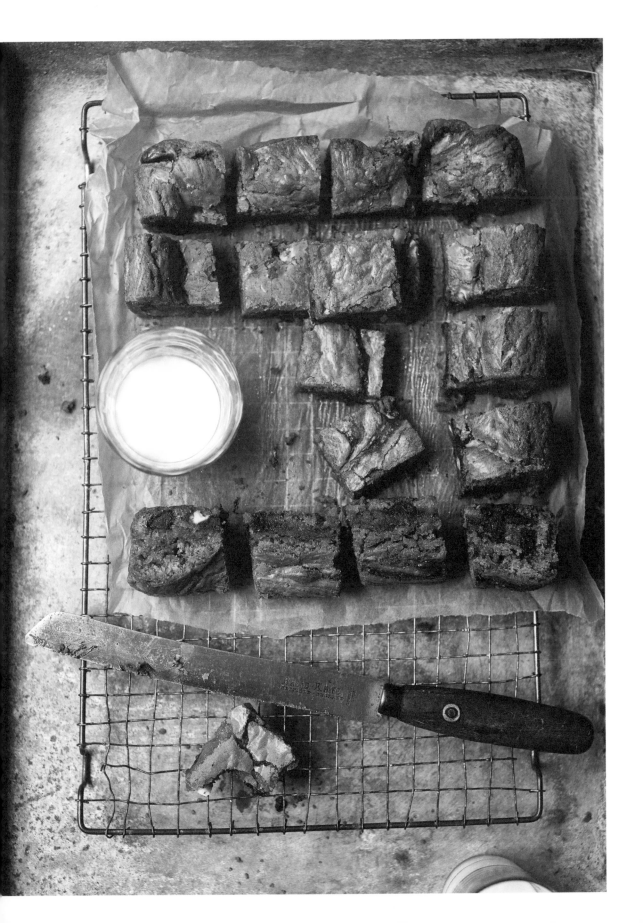

CHERRY BAKEWELL BUNDT

This familiar-flavoured cake has become a bit of a hit with our (small) book team, who single-handedly polished off the entire thing in a day. It is subtle in flavour and has a wonderfully smooth texture. It also keeps really well for a few days when stored in a cake tin/airtight container, which is always a winner; stale cakes are upsetting. So, this is for Isla and Kendal and Laura, who seem to love this cake more than anything else.

SERVES 16
—

250g unsalted butter, at room temperature, plus extra for greasing

350g plain flour, plus extra for the tin

150g fresh cherries

75g maraschino cherries, or glacé cherries

500g caster sugar

6 large eggs

½ teaspoon good-quality almond extract

¼ teaspoon fine salt

2 teaspoons baking powder

300ml milk

75g ground almonds

2 tablespoons flaked almonds

200g icing sugar

2 tablespoons amaretto *(or just use water)*

Start by preheating your oven to 180°C/gas 4. Grease your bundt tin with butter (I use a pastry brush to get into all the nooks and crannies), then liberally dust with flour and shake out the excess.

Remove the stones from the fresh cherries, blitz in a food processor with the maraschino cherries until you have a purée, then leave to one side. In a free-standing mixer, or by hand using some elbow grease, beat together the butter and sugar until it is pale and light. Gradually beat in the eggs, followed by the almond extract and salt. Beat in half the flour and baking powder, just enough to combine, followed by the milk. Gently fold in the remaining flour and baking powder with a large metal spoon, and finish by folding in the ground almonds.

Spoon one third of the cake mixture into your bundt tin, then evenly spoon over a third of the cherry purée, gently rippling it into the batter. Repeat twice, so both mixtures are used up, then pop the tin into the oven and bake for around 50 minutes – 1 hour, until your cake is golden and cooked through. Leave to cool in the tin for 15 minutes, then turn out on to a rack to cool completely.

While the cake is cooling, scatter the flaked almonds on a baking tray and pop them into the oven for 3–4 minutes, until golden. Leave to one side to cool. When you are ready to decorate, sift the icing sugar into a bowl and stir in just enough amaretto to make a thick icing. Drizzle it over the cake, and scatter over the toasted flaked almonds.

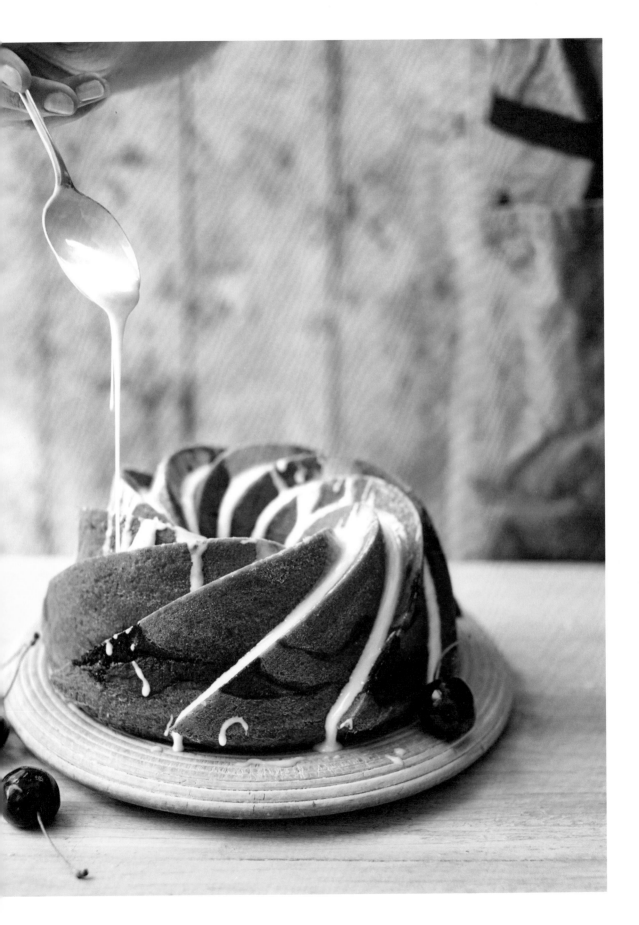

MY FAVOURITE CITRUS CAKE

Being an avid cake maker, I am oftened asked what my favourite cake is. And it has to be a cross between a classic lemon drizzle cake and a lemon poppy seed cake. I want poppy seeds and I want drizzle. Not the most flamboyant recipe, but it's my favourite, and it's screaming out for a natter with your mates or a trip to your nan's.

SERVES 8–10
—

200g unsalted butter, at room temperature, plus extra for greasing

2 heaped tablespoons poppy seeds

2 tablespoons milk

400g golden caster sugar

3 lemons *(you can use other citrus if you like – I like to replace some of the lemons with blood orange or bergamot when they're in season)*

½ a vanilla pod

4 large eggs

200g self-raising flour

Preheat your oven to 170°C/gas 3. Grease a 1 litre loaf tin and line with greaseproof paper.

Mix the poppy seeds and milk together in a small bowl and leave to one side.

Place the butter in the bowl of a free-standing mixer and beat for a couple of minutes, then add 200g of the golden caster sugar. Beat for a further 2–3 minutes, or until you have a pale and fluffy mixture. (You can of course do this with an electric mixer, or by hand using a little elbow grease.) Finely grate in the zest of the lemons, scrape in the seeds from the vanilla pod, and beat everything together well.

Beat the eggs in, one at a time, until they have all been incorporated. Sift in the flour, and stir into the cake batter with a large metal spoon, keeping the mixture as light as possible. Finally stir in the milk and poppy seeds, then spoon the cake batter into the prepared tin. Sprinkle over 30g of caster sugar, then pop the tin into the oven and bake for 45–50 minutes, or until golden and cooked through.

While the cake is cooking, make the drizzle. Squeeze the juice from the lemons into a small pan and stir in the remaining 170g of golden caster sugar. Pop the pan on a medium heat and cook for around 4–5 minutes, until the sugar has dissolved and you have a thick syrup. Leave to one side to cool.

When the cake is ready, leave it in the tin for 5 minutes before placing it on a cooling rack. Pierce the top of the cake repeatedly and evenly with a skewer, then drizzle over the cooled syrup. Leave the cake to cool completely, and serve.

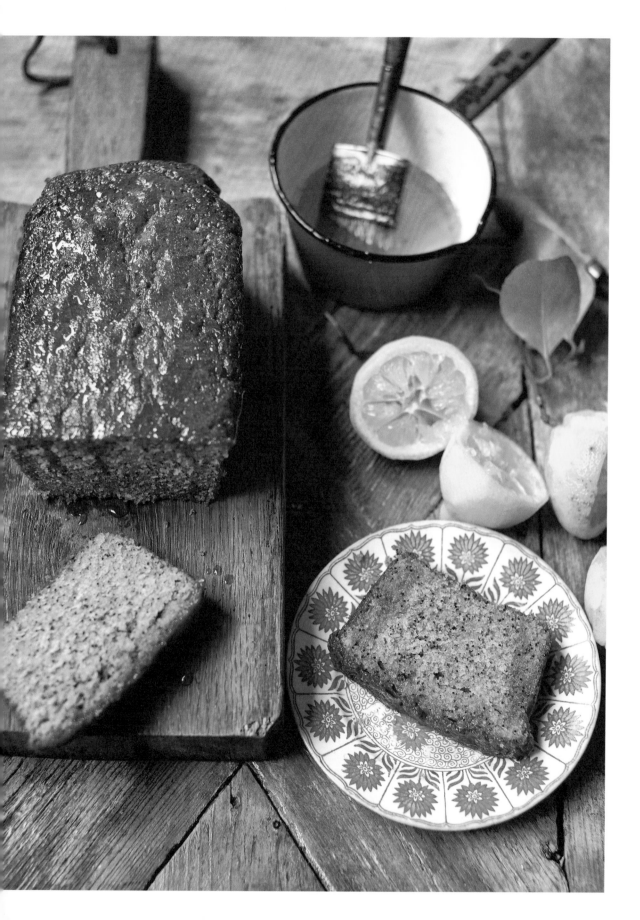

PRALINE ORCHARD PIE WITH BOURBON

As I mentioned in a previous chapter, I just don't think you can go wrong with a pie. They are perfect for times when you want to zone out, unwind and put your focus on just one thing. They're also such a wonderful gift: no one can say no to a pie. And this recipe is worthy of all that – it's familiar but has been taken up a notch. The hazelnutty pastry and crunchy praline top give it a fantastic edge, and don't be put off by the bourbon – it cooks away but leaves the pie with a gorgeous caramel richness.

SERVES 8
—

100g hazelnuts

250g cold unsalted butter, plus extra for greasing

440g plain flour, plus extra for dusting

50g icing sugar

1 large egg

75ml bourbon or whisky

a good pinch of sea salt

750g Bramley apples

300g firm pears

½ lemon

125g light soft brown sugar

125g granulated sugar

1 teaspoon ground cinnamon

½ teaspoon mixed spice

1 fresh bay leaf

75ml milk

proper custard, to serve *(see page 245)*

Blitz 60g of the hazelnuts in a food processor until you have a fine powder. Cut 200g of the butter into cubes. Sift 400g of flour into a large bowl with the ground hazelnuts and icing sugar, then rub in the cubes of butter until the mixture resembles breadcrumbs (alternatively you can do this in a food processor). Beat the egg with 50ml of bourbon (or whisky) and a pinch of salt, and mix most of it into the butter and flour until you have a ball of dough – be careful not to work it too much. Reserve the unused egg mixture to brush the pie lid later. Lightly flour the dough, wrap it in clingfilm and chill in the fridge for 1 hour.

While your pastry is chilling, preheat your oven to 180°C/gas 4. Peel the apples and pears and cut them into 2½cm chunks. Put all the fruit into a big bowl and toss with the juice from the lemon half then leave to one side.

In another bowl whisk together 50g of the granulated sugar, all of the soft light brown sugar, the remaining 40g of flour, the cinnamon and the mixed spice.

Put the remaining 40g of hazelnuts on a baking tray and pop into the oven for 6–8 minutes, until golden and toasted. Remove from the tray (but do not turn the oven off), leave to cool and then roughly chop. Grease a shallow 26cm pie dish with butter and leave to one side.

When the pastry and filling are ready, dust your worktop with a little flour and cut the pastry almost in half with one piece slightly larger. Roll out the larger of the pieces to ½cm thick, and line the base of the buttered pie dish. Mix the fruit with the sugar mixture and bay leaf and spoon into the pastry-lined pie dish. Brush the edges of the pie with a little milk, then roll out the second piece of pastry to 1cm thick and lay it over the top of »

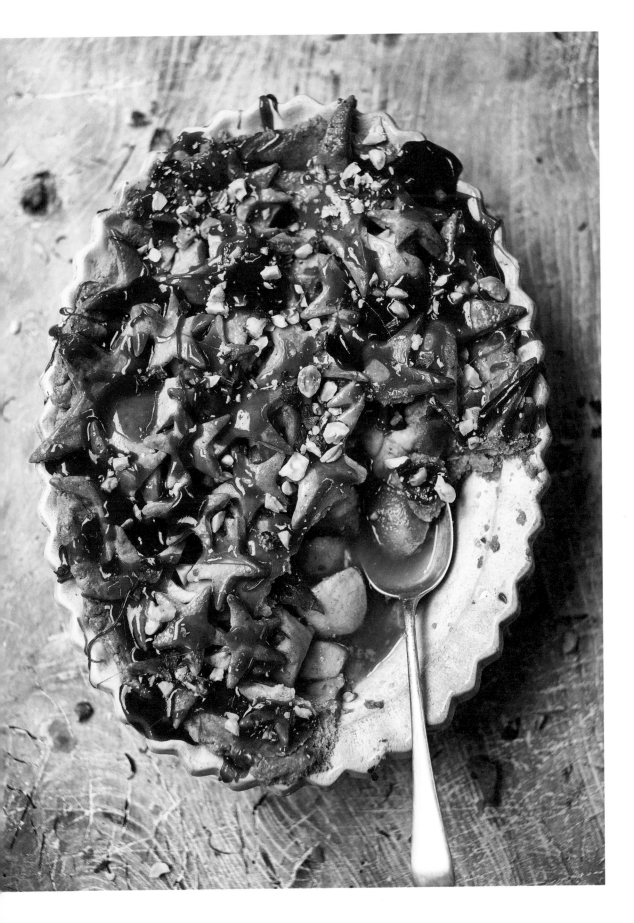

« the pie. Trim the excess edges, then, with your fingers, crimp together the edges of the pastry base and top. (Alternatively, use a cookie cutter to cut your chosen shapes out of the pastry and cover the pie with them.) Cut a slit in your pastry lid and brush the top of the pie with the remaining egg wash, then cover it with foil and place the dish directly at the bottom of your preheated oven. Bake for 30 minutes, then remove the foil and bake for a further 35–40 minutes, until golden on top.

When the pie is out of the oven, make the praline topping. Melt the remaining 50g of butter in a small saucepan with the remaining 75g of granulated sugar and 25ml of bourbon. Gently bring to the boil, then leave on a medium heat for 6–8 minutes, until you have a golden caramel. Make sure you swirl the pan rather than stir, otherwise the sugar will crystallise. Drizzle the caramel over the baked pie and scatter over the chopped toasted hazelnuts. Make sure you leave the pie to cool for at least 30 minutes, before serving to give the filling a chance to thicken, then serve with a large jug of vanilla bean custard or ice cream.

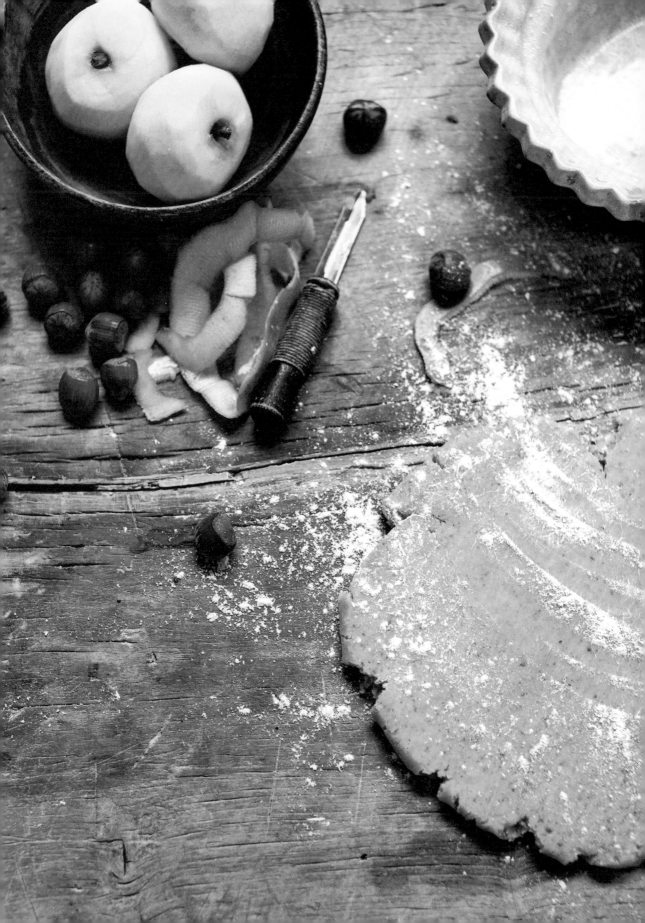

BRITISH SUMMERTIME STACK

I thought of a million names for this cake and none of them do it justice. If I could bottle up England in the summertime and bake it? This would be it. Think jugs of Pimm's in the sunshine, deckchairs, Wimbledon and bowls of Eton mess, all rolled into one. A sunny, crowd-pleasing number.

SERVES 10-12

—

150g butter, plus extra for greasing

490g caster sugar

5 large eggs

1 orange

1 lemon

150g self-raising flour

½ teaspoon baking powder

2-3 tablespoons milk

700g strawberries

125ml Pimm's, plus extra for brushing

200ml double cream

1 vanilla pod

200g fat-free Greek yoghurt

icing sugar, to serve

fresh mint leaves or flowers, for decorating *(optional)*

Preheat the oven to 180°C/gas 4. Grease two 20cm round cake tins and line with greaseproof paper.

Cream the butter and 150g of sugar in a free-standing mixer until pale. Separate the eggs, and add the yolks to the mixer (keeping the whites to one side for later). Finely grate in the zest of the orange and lemon and beat. Fold in the flour and baking powder, followed by enough milk to give you a smooth, creamy batter. Evenly divide the batter between the tins and spread out. Don't worry if it doesn't look enough – it will be, I promise. Pop the tins into the oven and bake the cakes for 25 minutes, until golden and cooked through. Leave to cool in the tins for 5 minutes, then transfer to a rack and leave to cool completely.

Reduce the oven temperature to 150°C/gas 2. In a clean bowl whisk the egg whites until soft peaks form, then slowly pour in 250g of caster sugar. Keep whisking for around 6 minutes, until the whites are glossy and stiff.

Cut two pieces of greaseproof paper, big enough to line two baking sheets, and draw around the cake tins with a pen. Turn the sheets over and lay them on the baking sheets, sticking them down in the corners with a little meringue. Divide the meringue between the two circles (you should be able to see the outline faintly through the paper) and spread it out so it is just within the circles – the meringue will spread a little as it cooks. Smooth the top of one of the meringue discs and peak the other with the back of a spoon to give you a pointy texture – this will be the top. Bake for around 70 minutes, until cooked through but not too dry. Leave to cool on the baking sheets.

While the meringues are cooling, make the fruit filling. Hull and chop 500g of the strawberries and place in a small pan with the Pimm's and the remaining 90g of sugar. Bring to the boil, then reduce the heat a little and »

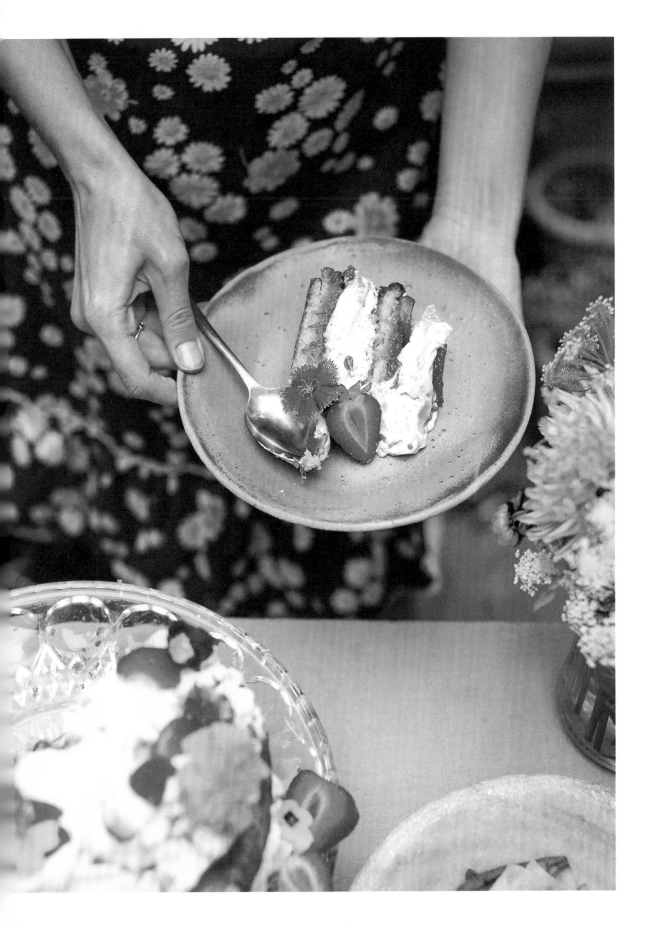

« leave to bubble away for 8–10 minutes until you have a sticky strawberry Pimm's compote. Leave to cool. Hull, quarter and slice the remaining 200g strawberries.

When you are ready to layer your cakes, whisk the cream until soft peaks form, scrape in the vanilla seeds, and fold in the yoghurt. Place one of the sponges on a board or cake stand and brush with a spoonful of Pimm's. Drizzle over half the strawberry compote and top with the un-peaked meringue. Spoon over most of the vanilla cream and most of the sliced strawberries. Top with the second sponge, brush with another spoonful of Pimm's and most of the remaining compote, and add the final peaked meringue layer.

Top with a few dollops of the cream mixture, a drizzle of strawberry compote and the remaining sliced strawberries. Sieve over a little icing sugar and decorate with mint leaves and edible flowers, if you like.

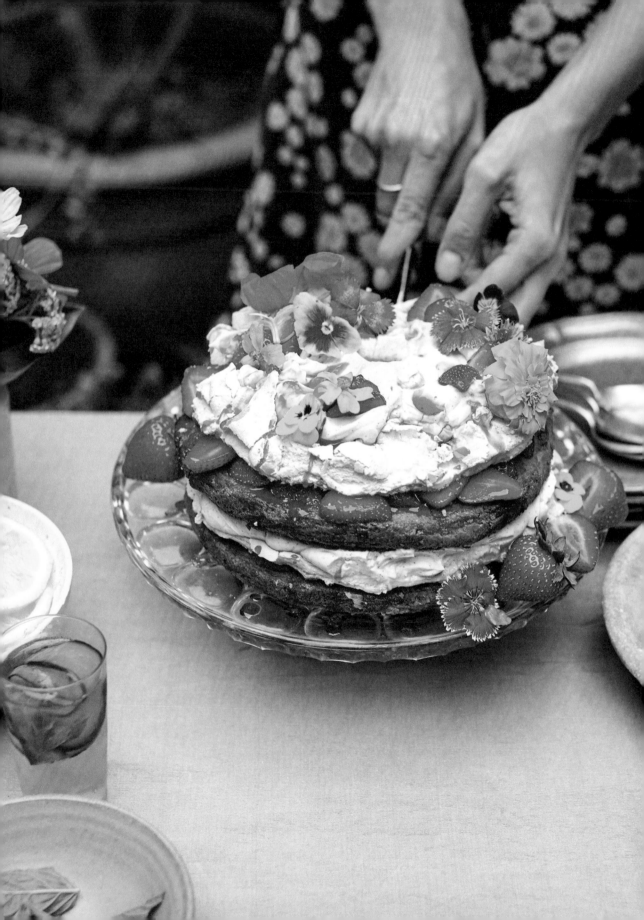

BANANA CAKE WITH PEANUT BUTTER FROSTING

This cake started out as a gift for my dentist and it got everyone talking – presumably because of the sugar content for a dentist. However, I can report back that they loved it, and not a filling in sight. I've made it a few times since and it's a total winner; my entire family love it and they're a tough bunch to please. It's a great 'gift' cake, as it keeps really well and stays moist for a few days.

SERVES 10–12

—

150ml olive oil *(or other flavourless oil)*

½ tablespoon good-quality vanilla extract

2 large eggs

75g natural yoghurt

4 large or 5 medium very ripe bananas

a squeeze of lemon juice

100g soft dark brown sugar

60g caster sugar

200ml milk

225g wholemeal or plain flour

1 teaspoon baking powder

1 teaspoon bicarbonate of soda

a good pinch of fine sea salt

125g butter, at room temperature

125g smooth peanut butter *(or almond butter works wonderfully too)*

250g icing sugar

3 tablespoons maple syrup

Preheat your oven to 180°/gas 4. Line a 1 litre loaf tin with greaseproof paper and leave to one side.

In a large mixing bowl, whisk together the olive oil, vanilla, eggs and yoghurt. Mash the bananas in a separate bowl with a squeeze of lemon juice. Mash in the dark brown and caster sugars, then whisk into the oil mixture and add 150ml of the milk. Sift the flour, baking powder, bicarbonate of soda and salt into the bowl, and tip in any roughage from the flour that's left in the sieve (if using wholemeal). Fold into the banana mixture with a large metal spoon and pour into the lined loaf tin.

Pop the tin into the middle of the oven and bake for around 50 minutes, until the cake is cooked through. Check with a skewer, but be prepared for a little residue, as the cake is naturally quite damp. However, if it still looks a little raw, pop it back into the oven for a further 10 minutes.

Leave the cake to cool in the tin for around 10 minutes, then remove from the tin and transfer to a rack to cool completely.

While the cake is cooling, make the buttercream. Beat the butter and peanut butter in a free-standing mixer (or with an electric hand whisk) for a few minutes until pale and creamy. Sift in the icing sugar, add 25ml of milk and beat for a further 5 minutes, until incredibly pale and smooth. If it still feels a little thick beat in the remaining 25ml of milk, then ripple in 2 tablespoons of maple syrup.

Once the cake is cool, spread it with the peanut butter frosting, drizzle on the remaining maple syrup and it's ready to go.

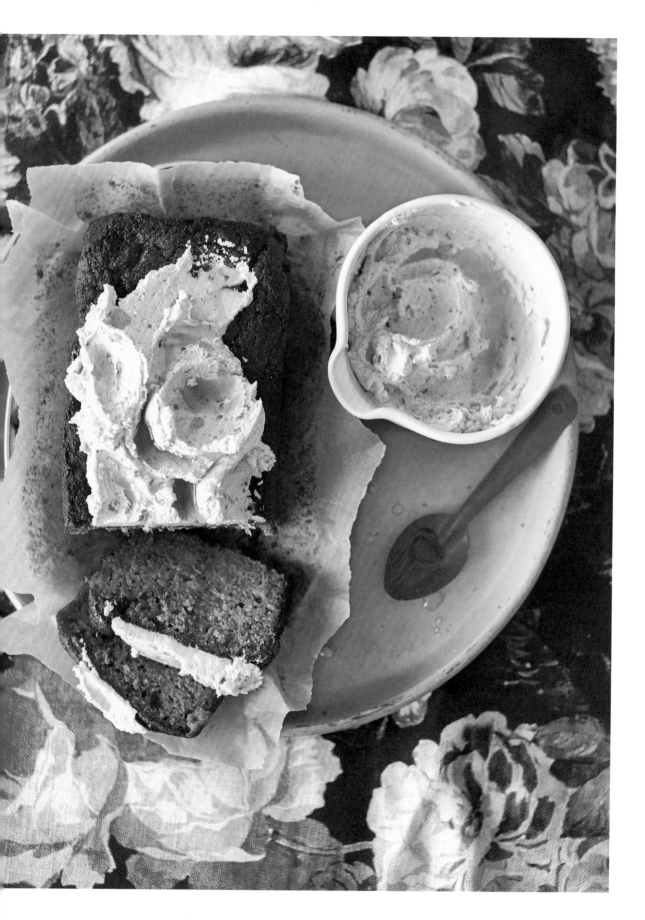

PUMPKIN AND GINGER LAYER CAKE

If you like carrot cake then this is for you – damp, spiced and delicious. The use of yoghurt and puréed pumpkin gives this sponge a velvety smooth yet light texture.

SERVES 16
—

4 large eggs

250ml olive oil

1 teaspoon vanilla extract

100g natural yoghurt

250g caster sugar

150g soft light brown sugar

300g puréed pumpkin *(see instructions on page 214)*

475g plain flour

2 heaped teaspoons ground cinnamon

1 teaspoon mixed spice

2 teaspoons baking powder

1 teaspoon bicarbonate of soda

a pinch of sea salt

a little spiced rum, for brushing

FOR THE FROSTING
—

40g pumpkin seeds

500g icing sugar

250g butter, at room temperature

200g cream cheese

3 balls of stem ginger

Preheat the oven to 180°C/gas 4. Grease two 20cm springform cake tins and line the bases with greaseproof paper.

In a large mixing bowl whisk together the eggs, olive oil, vanilla, yoghurt, caster and soft light brown sugars and the pumpkin purée until you have a smooth mixture. Into another bowl, sift the flour, ground cinnamon, mixed spice, baking powder, bicarbonate of soda and salt, then fold into the pumpkin batter. Divide evenly between the two tins and bake on the middle shelf of your oven for around 45 minutes, or until cooked through. Check with a skewer – it should come out clean. If the cakes are still a little raw, bake for a further 5–10 minutes. Leave the sponges to cool in the tins for 5 minutes, then transfer to a rack to cool completely.

While the oven is still on, caramelise the pumpkin seeds for the frosting. Rinse them in a sieve, then toss them in 1 heaped tablespoon of the icing sugar until lightly coated. Spread out on a baking sheet and pop into the oven for 10 minutes, until caramelised and crunchy. Remove and leave to one side to cool.

While the cakes are cooling, make your frosting. Cut the butter into cubes and put them into a free-standing mixer with a paddle attachment (or just use a large mixing bowl and handheld mixer if you don't have one). Beat for 3–4 minutes, until pale and light. Drain any excess liquid from the cream cheese and beat into the butter, only just enough to mix the two together – too much and it becomes runny. Sift half the remaining icing sugar into the mix, and when fully combined sift and beat in the remaining half. Keep beating for around 4 minutes, until pale and smooth. Finely chop the stem ginger and add it to the frosting with a little of the syrup from the jar. Place the bowl of frosting in the fridge for 30 minutes to firm up.

When the sponges have cooled completely, carefully cut them in half horizontally and layer them up on your serving board or cake stand with the cream cheese frosting, brushing the layers with a little spiced rum as »

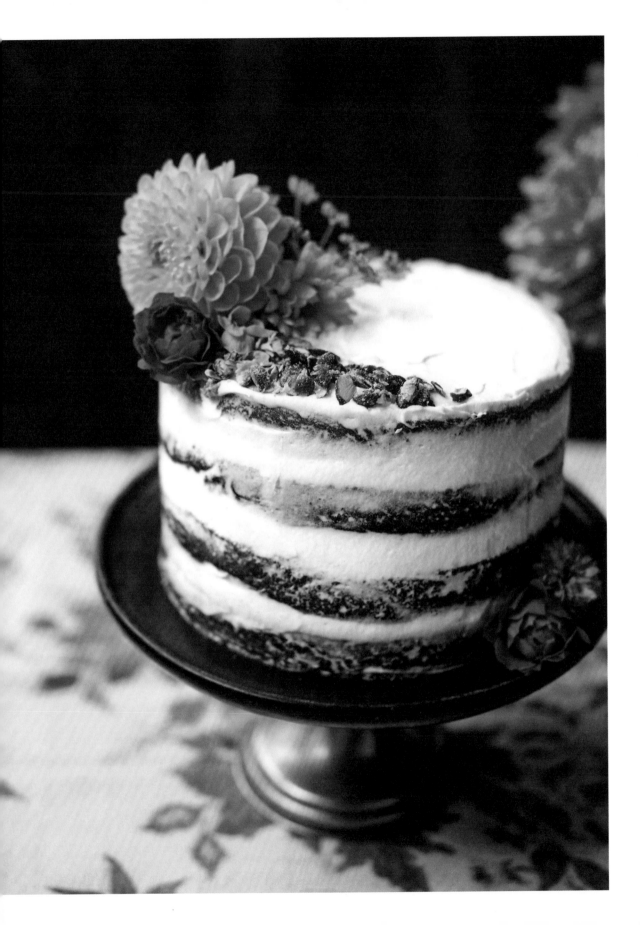

« you go. You can leave the cake like that, or use the last bit of frosting to give your cake a scant frosting around the sides and top. Decorate with the caramelised seeds, and pop back into the fridge for at least 30 minutes before serving – just to give the frosting time to firm up.

TO MAKE THE PUMPKIN PURÉE
—

Peel around 400g of pumpkin or squash and cut into chunks. Boil until cooked through. Drain and leave to cool, then blitz in a food processor with just enough water to make a purée.

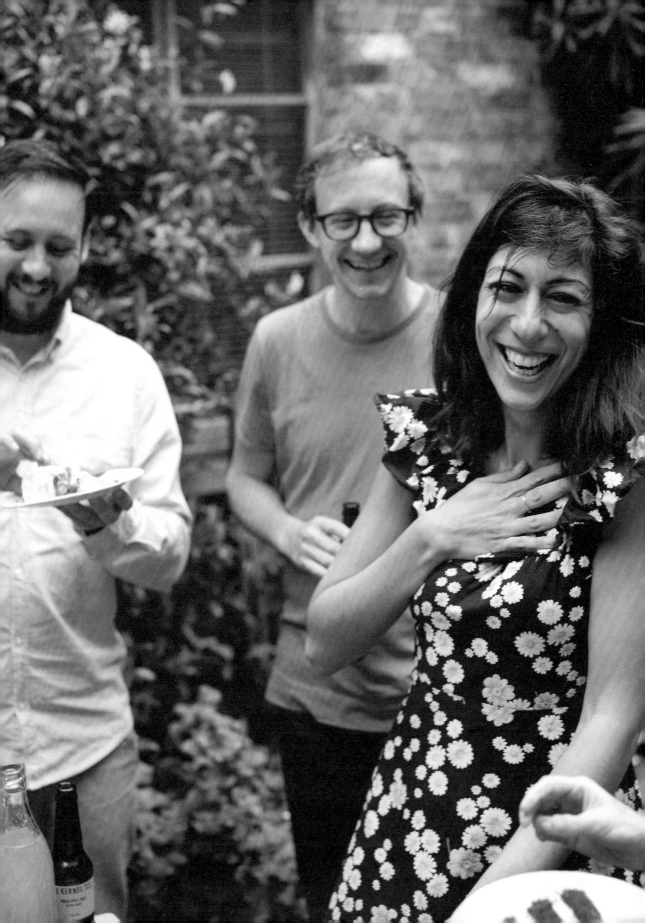

CREAMY RICE PUDDING WITH SHERRY AND ROSEMARY POACHED PRUNES

This recipe is pure nostalgia. I'm sure I'm not the only one who grew up eating baked rice pudding and tinned prunes in the '80s. Gone, however, are the syrupy, painfully sweet prunes. And in their place are prunes poached with bay, rosemary and sherry and blitzed to a flavour-packed purée. Rippled into creamy, risotto-esque rice pudding, this is homely comfort food at its best.

SERVES 6
—

1 orange

100g pitted prunes

1 fresh bay leaf

1 sprig of rosemary

60ml dry oloroso sherry

4 tablespoons soft light brown sugar

1 litre full-fat or semi-skimmed milk

175g pudding rice

a good pinch of sea salt

150ml double cream

Finely grate the orange zest and keep to one side. Place the prunes, bay leaf, rosemary and sherry in a small pan. Add 2 tablespoons of the soft light brown sugar and 2 tablespoons of water. Pop the pan on a medium heat and gently bring to the boil. As soon as it starts to bubble up, reduce the heat to low and leave to simmer for 5 minutes, until lightly syrupy. Remove the pan from the heat and leave to cool.

Once completely cool, pour the prunes and syrup into a food processor and squeeze in the orange juice. Blitz until completely smooth, adding a splash of water if it is a little thick, then spoon into a bowl. You are looking for a thick but spoonable texture. Alternatively, just keep the prunes whole – my mum loves them like that.

Pour the milk into a large saucepan with the pudding rice, and place on a medium-high heat. Bring to the boil, give it a good stir, then cover with a lid and reduce the heat to low. Leave to gently cook for 20 minutes, stirring occasionally. Remove the lid and cook for a final 5 minutes, stirring it almost constantly, until rich and creamy. Stir in the salt, the remaining 2 tablespoons of sugar and the double cream, and remove from the heat.

Ladle the rice pudding into bowls and ripple through the puréed prunes. Finish by sprinkling over the grated orange zest, and serve.

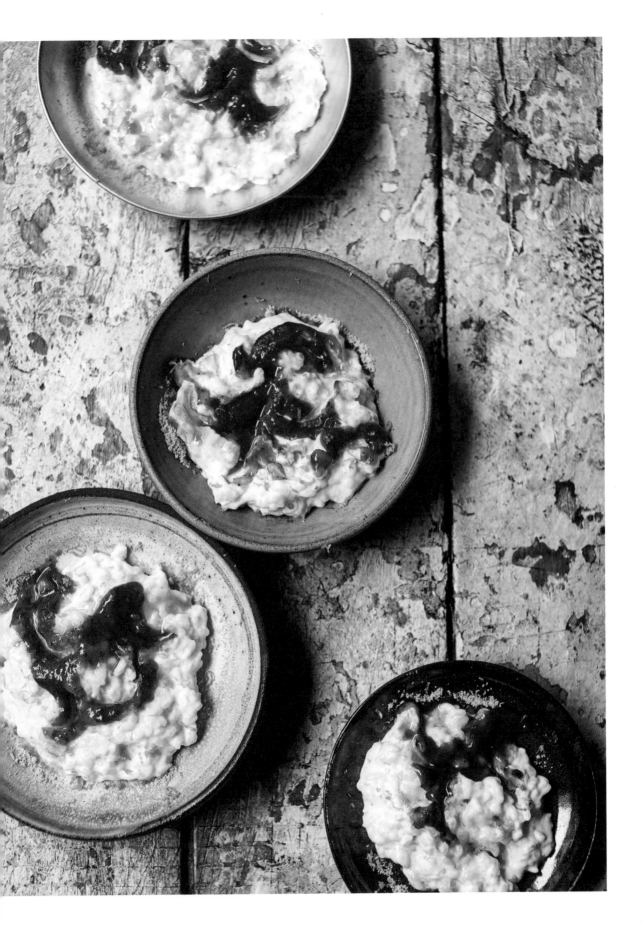

MALTED MILK CHOCOLATE AND RASPBERRY TART

This tart is inspired by a combination of treats we had as kids: malted biscuits, milky hot chocolate and sticky homemade jam tarts. It requires a little time and patience but manages to be both elegant and comforting at the same time. You could of course serve it for pud at a dinner party, finished with a few fresh berries, a dollop of crème fraîche and a delicious dessert wine – however, for me it is just screaming for a glass of milk and a blanket.

SERVES 16

—

125g cold unsalted butter

250g plain flour, plus extra for dusting

40g icing sugar

3 tablespoons malt powder, such as Horlicks *(be sure not to use the 'light' kind)*

2 large eggs + 1 large egg yolk

200ml milk, plus a splash

200g raspberries *(you could use blackberries too)*

75g caster sugar

400ml double cream

400g good-quality milk chocolate, plus extra for serving

a good pinch of sea salt

Cut the butter into cubes. Sift the flour, icing sugar and 1 tablespoon of the malt powder into a large bowl, then rub in the cubes of butter until the mixture resembles breadcrumbs. Beat the egg yolk with a splash of milk and mix into the butter and flour until you have a ball of dough – be careful not to work it too much. Lightly flour the dough, wrap it in clingfilm and chill in the fridge for 30 minutes.

Roll the dough out on a clean floured surface until it's around 0.5cm thick. Loosely roll it around the rolling pin, then unroll it over a deep 25cm loose-bottomed tart tin. Ease the pastry into the tin, pushing it into the corners. Trim off any excess overhanging pastry, wrap that in clingfilm and keep it for later – you may need to patch up a little of the base once it's been blind baked. Prick the base of the tart all over with a fork. Cover with clingfilm and chill in the fridge for another 30 minutes.

While the pastry is chilling, preheat the oven to 180°C/gas 4. Next make the raspberry compote. Place 150g of the raspberries in a small saucepan and mix in the caster sugar. Mash them together and place on a medium-low heat. Bring it up to a light simmer, then leave to bubble away for around 6–8 minutes, so that you have a light jam. Leave to one side to cool completely.

Remove the clingfilm from the chilled base, then line it with scrunched-up greaseproof paper and fill with baking beans or uncooked rice. Blind bake for 12 minutes, then remove the paper and baking beans or rice and bake for a further 8–10 minutes, until lightly golden. When it is ready, take it out and turn down the oven to 150°C/gas 2.

Meanwhile, pour the cream and the 150ml of milk into a small pan and gently bring to the boil. Cut the chocolate into small pieces and place in a large mixing bowl. Just before the cream mixture starts to bubble, remove it from the heat and pour it over the chopped chocolate, adding a good pinch of sea salt. Leave it for a minute, then gently stir until completely smooth. Whisk the 2 eggs and beat into the chocolate cream with the remaining 2 tablespoons of malt powder.

Pop the blind baked case on to a baking sheet. Spoon the cooled raspberry jam into the case and spread it out to the edges. Pour over the chocolate cream and evenly scatter over the remaining raspberries. Place the tart in the oven and bake for 45–50 minutes, until the filling is just set and still has a little wobble. Leave to cool in the tin. When the tart is at room temperature and the filling is set, transfer to a serving plate or board. Finish by topping with the remaining raspberries and shavings of chocolate.

NECTARINE, CHAMOMILE AND HONEY GRANITA

Calming chamomile, ripe nectarines and only honey to sweeten: this recipe is a total winner in my eyes. It is subtle but delicious, and feels cleansing at the same time. If you have an ice cream machine you could churn it instead of shaving the ice, giving you a smooth and slightly sherbet-y sorbet.

SERVES 6

—

4 chamomile tea bags

100g honey

½ a lemon

750g nectarine

Place the chamomile tea bags in a small saucepan with 350ml of water and gently bring to the boil. As soon as it starts to bubble, remove from the heat and leave to one side to steep for 10 minutes. After 10 minutes remove the tea bags from the pan and stir in the honey. Pop the pan back on the hob, bring to the boil again, then leave to bubble away for 1 minute. Remove from the heat and leave to one side to cool completely.

When the chamomile honey syrup has cooled, pour it into a food processor and squeeze in the lemon juice. Roughly chop the nectarines, removing their stones, and add to the bowl. Blitz until smooth, then pour into your chosen container. Pop into the freezer and freeze for 3–4 hours. Use a fork to scrape the frozen granita, shaving the ice into the centre of the dish until it has all been scraped. Pop the dish back into the freezer for a further hour or two.

When you are ready to serve, remove the dish from the freezer and use a fork to scrape the granita into your serving bowls.

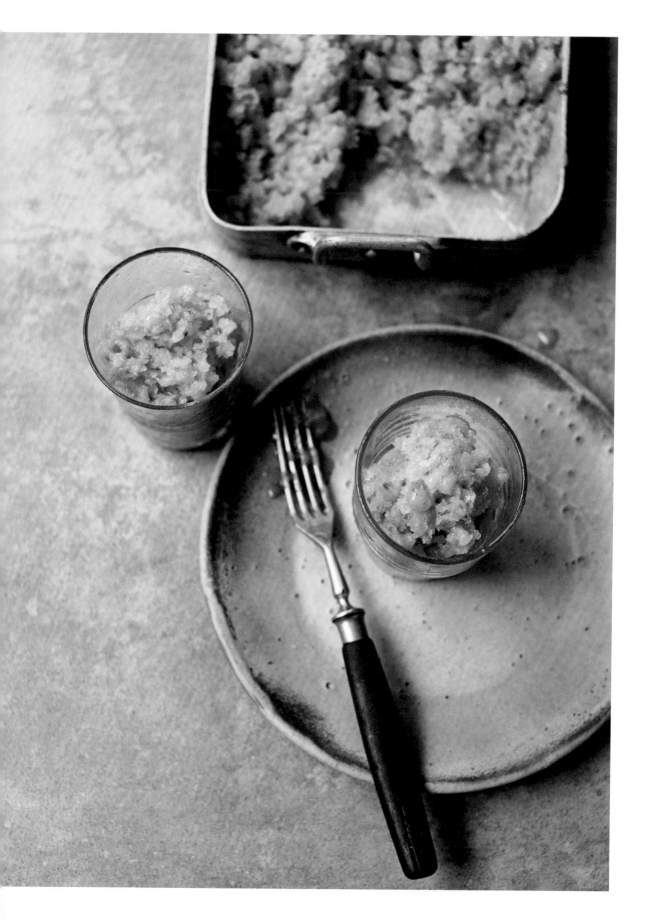

CHOCOLATE, RYE AND PECAN CELEBRATION CAKE

Everyone needs a cracking chocolate party cake up their sleeve and this is my current number one. I love the easiness of the sponge (melting and whisking, what a dream), which results in a dense fudgy texture, and the mixture of ground pecans and rye gives it a slight nuttiness too. Also, there's no denying that a cake this size, of many layers, gets people excited.

SERVES 16–20
—

600g butter, plus extra butter for greasing

150g pecans

125g dark chocolate, 70% cocoa solids

185g light soft brown sugar

225g caster sugar

a good pinch of sea salt

5 large eggs

1 teaspoon good-quality vanilla extract

150g wholemeal self-raising flour

100g rye flour

1¼ teaspoons baking powder

½ teaspoon bicarbonate of soda

500g icing sugar

a splash of milk

1 x sea salt caramel *(see page 246)*

edible gold dust or gold leaf *(optional)*

Grease a deep springform 20cm cake tin and line the base with greaseproof paper. Preheat the oven to 180°C/gas 4.

Place 75g of the pecans in a food processor and blitz until fine.

Put a large pan on a low heat and pour in 125ml of water. Dot in 250g of the butter and break in the chocolate. Add the light soft brown sugar, 75g of the caster sugar and a good pinch of salt. Melt over a low heat and whisk until smooth. As soon as it's ready, remove from the hob and leave to cool for 10 minutes before whisking in the eggs, vanilla and ground pecans.

In a large mixing bowl whisk together both the flours, the baking powder and bicarbonate of soda. Slowly pour in the hot chocolate mixture, whisking constantly until you have a smooth batter. Pour the mixture into the cake tin and pop into the oven for 55 minutes – 1 hour, or until cooked through. Leave to rest in the tin for 5 minutes, then transfer to a rack and leave to cool completely.

When your cake is cooled, slice it into three equal layers and leave to one side. If the top of your sponge is a little uneven, even it out and keep any sponge remnants for decorating later.

To make the caramel pecans, evenly sprinkle the remaining 150g of caster sugar into a large frying pan and place on a medium-low heat. Melt the sugar gently, swirling the pan to encourage it to melt evenly and never stirring it (this will form sugar crystals). Cover a baking sheet with greaseproof paper. As soon as the sugar has become a caramel, add the remaining pecans to the pan and quickly pour the hot pecan caramel on to the lined baking sheet. Leave to one side to cool. »

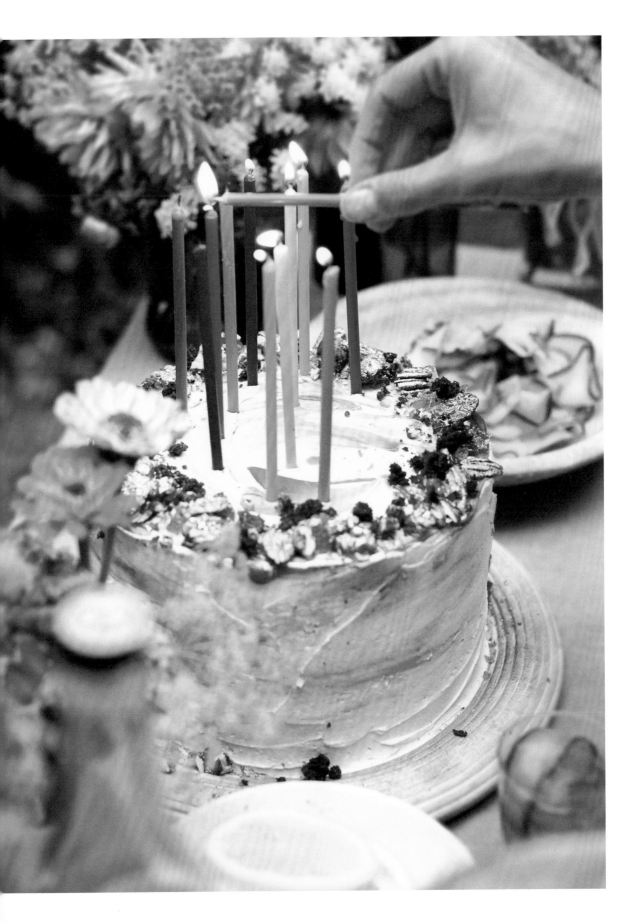

« Make the buttercream by beating the remaining 350g of butter in a free-standing mixer, or a bowl with an electric whisk, until pale and creamy. Sift in half the icing sugar and beat till smooth, then repeat with the remaining icing sugar. Continue to beat for a further 5 minutes until you have a pale and creamy buttercream. Beat in a splash of milk and one third of the sea salt caramel.

To layer your cake, dot a little buttercream on a cake stand or wooden board and place one of the layers on top (this will 'stick' it to the board). Spoon on a quarter of the buttercream and use a cake spatula to level it out. Drizzle with a little sea salt caramel and top with the second sponge. Repeat with a second layer of buttercream and caramel and top with the final sponge.

You can use the remaining buttercream to immediately cover the cakes, or, if you want a slightly slicker finish, try crumb-coating them first. To do this you'll need to apply a scant layer of buttercream to the top and sides of the cake, and use a cake spatula to scrape off any excess. The idea is you want just enough buttercream on there to 'catch' any loose crumbs. Doing this will also give you a great, even shape. Pop the cake into the fridge for 30–40 minutes to set the buttercream, then apply the final layer.

Finish the cake by drizzling any remaining sea salt caramel over the buttercream. For a slightly rippled effect, use a palette knife to work the sea salt caramel into the buttercream. Break the pecan caramel into pieces and dot around the edge of the cake, and crumble over any remnants of sponge. And for an even more opulent finish, dust the caramelised pecans with a little edible gold dust or leaf, if you like.

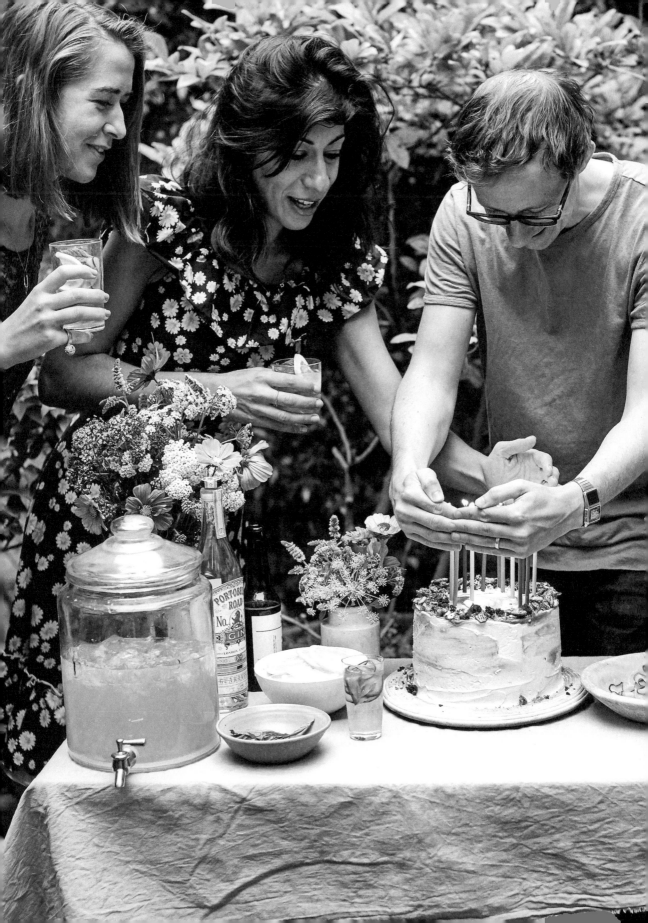

BLACK BREAD

Bread-making is a form of therapy in itself; there really is nothing quite like pummelling dough to get rid of unwanted stress and negative thoughts. And although there are a million recipes I could give you, I wanted to give you ones that are a little different while still being a fabulous way of unwinding. I wrote this black bread recipe for a Russian feature I was researching and instantly fell in love with it; so intense and complex. Laced with delicious spices and rich ingredients, it's a dense, sweet and heady bread. Please don't be put off the long ingredients list, it is totally worth the time and effort (and goes fantastically well with the cured salmon on page 40).

MAKES 1 LARGE LOAF
—

1 x 7g packet of fast-acting yeast

½ teaspoon caster sugar

2 tablespoons molasses

40g unsalted butter

a small shot of espresso

15g dark chocolate *(70% cocoa solids)*

½ shallot

½ tablespoon fennel seeds

200g wholemeal flour

200g rye flour

250g strong bread flour

70g bran

1 tablespoon sea salt

2 tablespoons cider vinegar

olive oil, for greasing

In a jug, mix the yeast and sugar with 100ml of tepid water and give it a good stir. Leave it to one side for 5–10 minutes, until the yeast activates and the surface becomes foamy.

In a pan, heat the molasses, butter, coffee and chocolate with 200ml of water, until the chocolate and butter have melted. Peel and finely chop the shallot. Grind the fennel seeds to a fine powder.

To knead the bread you can use an electric mixer with a paddle attachment, or do it by hand using a little elbow grease – I prefer by hand, far more therapeutic, and you can gauge the bread texture better. In your mixer or a large mixing bowl, whisk together all three flours, then scoop out about a third and leave it to one side. Mix the bran into the main bowl, along with the shallot, fennel seeds and salt then pour in the chocolate and yeast mixtures, and the cider vinegar. If you are using a mixer, put it on a medium speed and mix together until lovely and smooth, around 3–5 minutes. Otherwise use a wooden spoon to beat it by hand, although this will take a little longer.

Add the remaining flour a little at a time (reduce the speed if using a mixer), until it comes together into a dough. It should feel a little sticky, but firm and dense. You might not need all the flour; see how the dough feels. Turn it out on to a lightly floured surface and knead it well, for around 10 minutes, so it becomes springy and elastic. Mould the dough into a ball with your hands. Lightly grease a clean mixing bowl with olive oil and pop in the dough. Cover with a damp tea towel and leave it in a warm spot for around 2 hours, until it has doubled in size. »

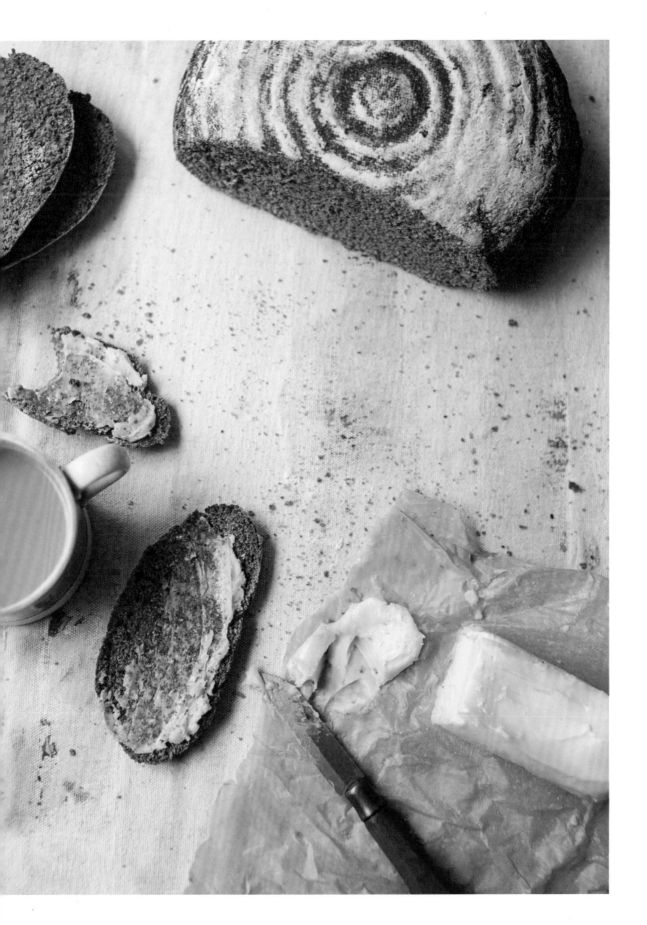

« Knock back the dough by turning it out on to a lightly floured surface and kneading for a couple of minutes. Form into a round loaf and place on a lightly greased baking tray, seam side down. Cover with a damp tea towel and leave to rise again for another couple of hours. Alternatively prove the dough in a floured bread-proving basket. While it is proving, preheat your oven to 180°C/gas 4.

When the bread is ready, place the tray in the oven for 50–60 minutes, or until browned on top and cooked through (if you are using a proving basket turn it on to a baking sheet first). The bread should sound hollow when knocked on the bottom. Serve with soft butter and anything you like – I love it with cured salmon.

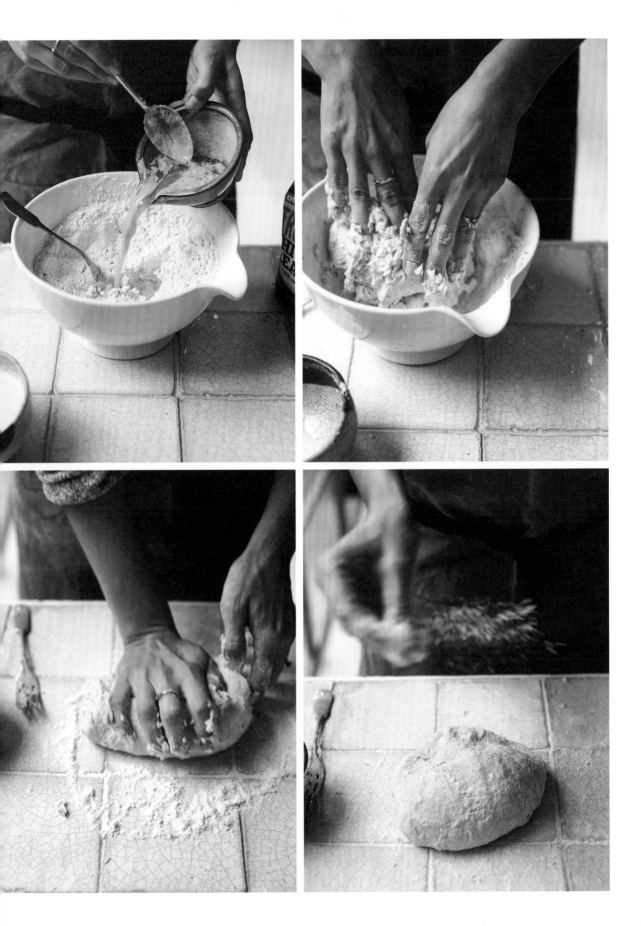

CARAWAY, HONEY AND BUTTERMILK BUNS

Growing up, my mum would occasionally treat us to mini brioche rolls from the local bakery after school, and fill them with strawberry jam. I loved the gentle sweetness and butteriness of the brioche, and in miniature form it felt so special. Twenty years of dreaming about those rolls, and my caraway, honey and buttermilk buns were created. Speckled with caraway seeds, these buns are wonderfully versatile – try them spread with apricot jam or filled with cheese. And if you're having a bad day, you could do worse than make a batch of these; kneading bread dough is more grounding than an hour-long yoga session. Cheaper too, I reckon.

MAKES 15 BUNS

—

3 tablespoons honey

1 x 7g packet of fast-acting yeast

60g unsalted butter

½ tablespoon caraway seeds

400g strong bread flour

1 teaspoon sea salt

250ml buttermilk

Olive oil, for greasing

1 egg yolk

Pour 75ml of warm water into a jug and stir in the honey and yeast. Leave to one side for 5 minutes. Melt the butter in a small pan. Crush the caraway seeds slightly in a mortar and pestle.

Mix the flour, caraway and salt in a large mixing bowl and make a well in the middle. Pour in the yeast mixture, buttermilk and butter and mix into the flour with a fork. Once it is all incorporated, turn the dough on to a well-floured surface and knead for 10 minutes, until you have a smooth and elastic dough. Try not to add too much flour, as this will make your dough dense; try to keep it a little damp. Form the dough into a ball. Lightly oil a large clean mixing bowl and pop in the dough to prove. Cover with a clean tea towel and leave it to rise in a draught-free warm spot for around 1–1½ hours. You want the dough to have doubled in size.

Turn the proved dough out on to your worktop and knock it back, kneading it for a few minutes. Roll the dough out and cut it into 15 even-sized pieces. Roll each piece into an even-sized ball and place in the tray you are going to bake them in. A tray around 25cm x 35cm works well, leaving a little room between the rolls so they can prove. Prove them again, covered with a tea towel, for a further 1–1½ hours, until doubled in size. Preheat your oven to 180°C/gas 4.

When the rolls have risen, whisk the egg yolk with a splash of water and brush the tops of the buns lightly. Pop the tray into the preheated oven for 18–20 minutes. The buns should be beautifully golden, and sound hollow when tapped underneath – this is how to check they are cooked through. Leave to cool, then serve.

—

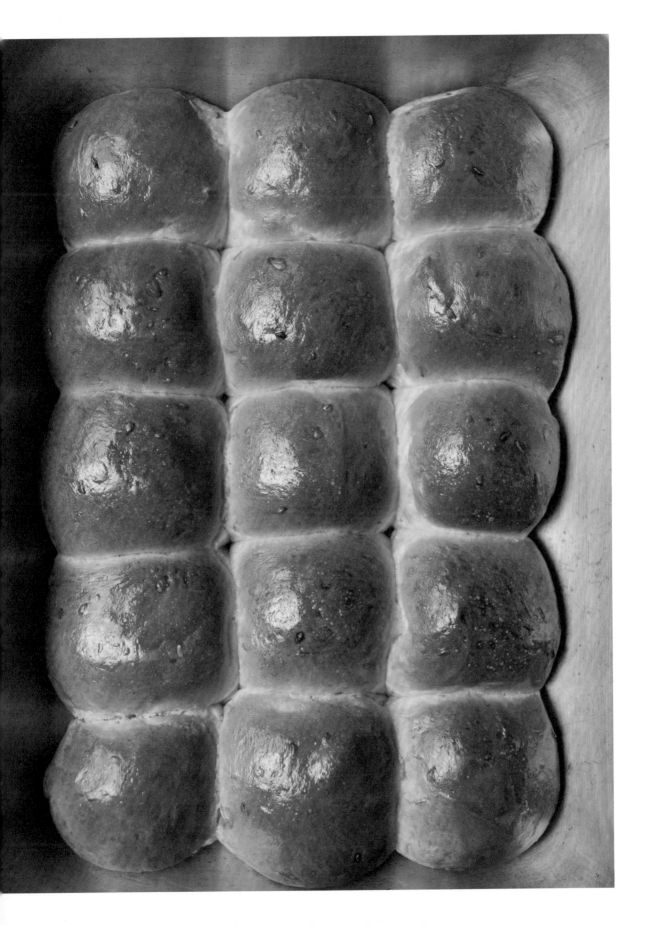

NO-CHURN CHAI ICE CREAM

The chai flavour here works perfectly with the sweetened milk, reminiscent of the condensed milk chai you get in India. Making the condensed milk from scratch takes a little time and patience but is perfect if, like me, you don't own an ice cream machine. Alternatively you can use the ready-made tinned stuff and it'll take less than 30 minutes to get the ice cream into the freezer.

MAKES 1 LITRE
—

1.25 litres full-fat milk *(or 397g tin of condensed milk and cut the sugar)*

300g golden granulated sugar

10 green cardamom pods

4 chai tea bags

1 cinnamon stick

¼ teaspoon ground ginger

6 cloves

a pinch of black pepper

500ml double cream

FOR THE CASHEW BRITTLE
—

200g caster sugar

100g cashew nuts

1 heaped tablespoon black or white sesame seeds

sea salt

gold leaf, optional

Place 1 litre of the milk in a large heavy-based saucepan, along with the sugar, and pop on to a medium-low heat. (It's vital to use a heavy-based pan, otherwise the milk will burn easily.) Cook the milk for 2 hours, stirring every 5–10 minutes with a heatproof spatula so that it doesn't catch on the bottom. When it has thickened and reduced by about half, remove from the heat and cover with a tea towel. Leave to cool.

While your condensed milk is ticking away, crush the cardamom pods and place in a small pan with 2 of the tea bags, all the other spices and the remaining 250ml of milk. Gently bring the milk to the boil, then reduce to a simmer for 5 minutes. Remove from the heat and leave to cool completely before straining. If you are using ready-made condensed milk, this is where you'll need to start the recipe.

When the infused and condensed milks have both completely cooled, pour them into a mixing bowl and pour in the cream. Cut open the remaining 2 tea bags and empty the leaves into the bowl. Whisk with an electric whisk until stiff peaks form, then spoon the mixture into your chosen dish and pop into the freezer for at least 6 hours. Take the dish out 10 minutes before you want to serve, so it has a chance to soften slightly. I like to serve the chai ice cream straight up, with crushed cashew brittle.

To make the brittle, line a baking sheet with greaseproof paper and pour the sugar into a large non-stick frying pan. Place on a medium heat and leave it to melt without stirring, swirling to encourage it along. When the sugar has completely melted, scatter in the cashews, sesame seeds and a good pinch of salt. Swirl to completely coat, then pour on to the greaseproof paper. Leave to cool and set, then bash with a rolling pin to crush. I like to press larger pieces of brittle with gold leaf, for a little Indian-inspired decadence.

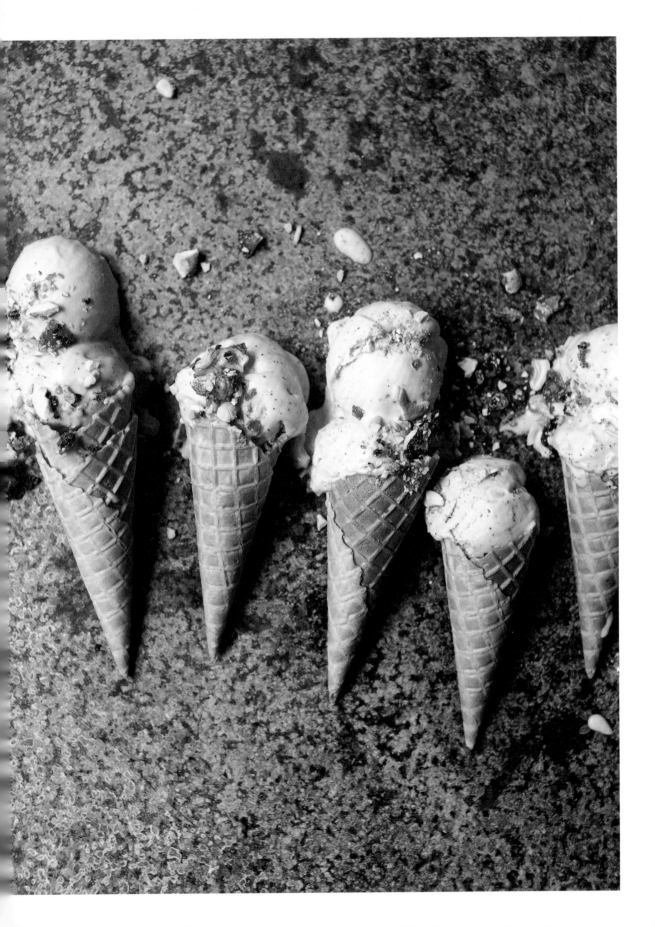

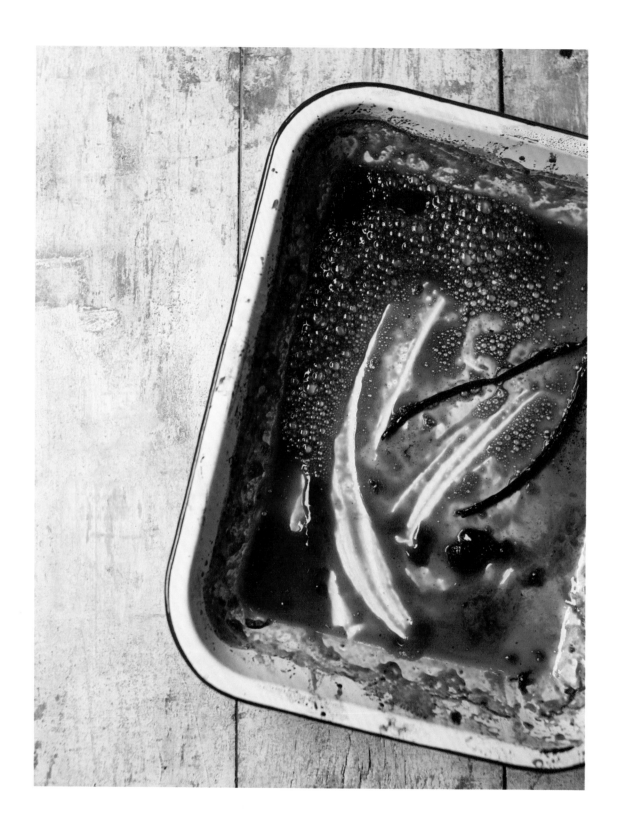

A BIT ON THE SIDE

—

And the final chapter, for all those extra things
that make everything taste better, but need
a bit of time and love. Homemade butter,
yoghurt, stocks, jams, chutneys, and even
delicious calming teas and infusions for the
end of the cooking day.

HOMEMADE YOGHURT

Making yoghurt is incredibly satisfying to do, and one of the first things my yiayia taught me. I've altered it slightly from how she makes hers, mostly because she seems to have an innate yoghurt-making ability and doesn't use a thermometer. So for consistency's sake I'm giving you temperatures. It might seem strange to buy yoghurt in order to make yoghurt, but like making bread you need a starter, and once you've made your own you can use your homemade yoghurt as the starter for the next batch.

MAKES 1 LITRE
—

1 litre full-fat milk, organic if possible

2 tablespoons milk powder (optional, but worth adding as it will give you a creamier yoghurt)

6 tablespoons natural live yoghurt, organic if possible

Start by sterilising your jars – if you haven't got one large jar, use a couple of medium-size ones. Wash the jars and lids thoroughly in hot soapy water, rinsing them well, then place them on a baking tray lined with baking paper. Make sure the jars aren't touching each other and pop them into a preheated oven, at 140°C/gas 1, for around 10 minutes. If you're using a Kilner jar, sterilise the rubber seals by soaking them in boiling water. Keep the oven on while you make the yoghurt.

Pour the milk into a large heavy-based saucepan and place on a medium heat. Once it reaches 82°C, remove from the heat immediately – don't let the milk come to the boil. Whisk in the milk powder and leave to one side for the temperature to drop. At this point turn off your oven. When the milk gets to 45°C, whisk in the yoghurt, then carefully ladle or spoon into the jars. You want to keep the jars warm for around 5–6 hours for the yoghurt to ferment. You can do this by wrapping them in tea towels and storing them in a warm cupboard, or you can do what I do and put them back into the turned-off, warm oven. After 5–6 hours you will have a thickened and tart yoghurt. Place the jars in the fridge for the yoghurt to thicken even more. It'll be ready after 3 hours.

Alternatively, you can cultivate the yoghurt in a heated thermos (you'll need a couple for this recipe, or you can just halve the quantities). Heat your thermos by filling it with almost boiling water and leaving it in there for 5 minutes. Carefully pour out the water and spoon in the yoghurt. Leave the yoghurt for 7–8 hours in the thermos, then pour into the sterilised jars and store in the fridge. Again, leave for 3 hours to set before eating.

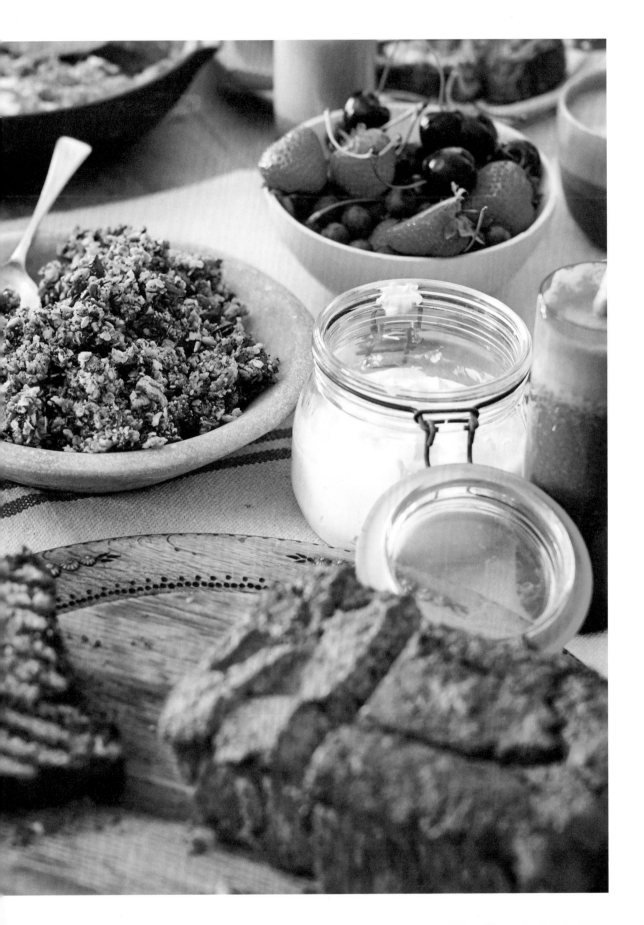

LABNEH

A simple way to make cheese at home, labneh is a beautifully mild Middle Eastern cream cheese that requires little effort. It is perfect as part of a meze or breakfast spread or even with fruit and honey as a pud. Incredibly simple and satisfying to make.

MAKES 1KG
—

1kg Greek yoghurt

2 teaspoons sea salt

In a large bowl mix together the yoghurt and sea salt. Line a sieve with a large double-layer piece of muslin and spoon in the salted yoghurt. Gather together the muslin sides and tie them together. Hang the yoghurt-filled muslin from a shelf in the fridge, with a bowl underneath to catch the whey. If you don't have bars to tie it to, try suspending it from a wooden spoon balanced on two large items. You could pop the sieve over a mixing bowl and place a plate with a weight on top of it (such as a heavy jar or tin), but gravity does give you a slightly superior, creamy labneh.

Leave the yoghurt draining for 24 hours, then remove from the muslin and serve. Made this way, labneh will keep for a couple of weeks in the fridge, in an airtight container. To store your labneh for longer, leave the yoghurt hanging for 36 hours, then roll the cheese into balls and carefully place in a sterilised jar (see page 238). Pour in enough olive oil to completely cover and pop into the fridge. Your labneh will keep for weeks, even months, this way.

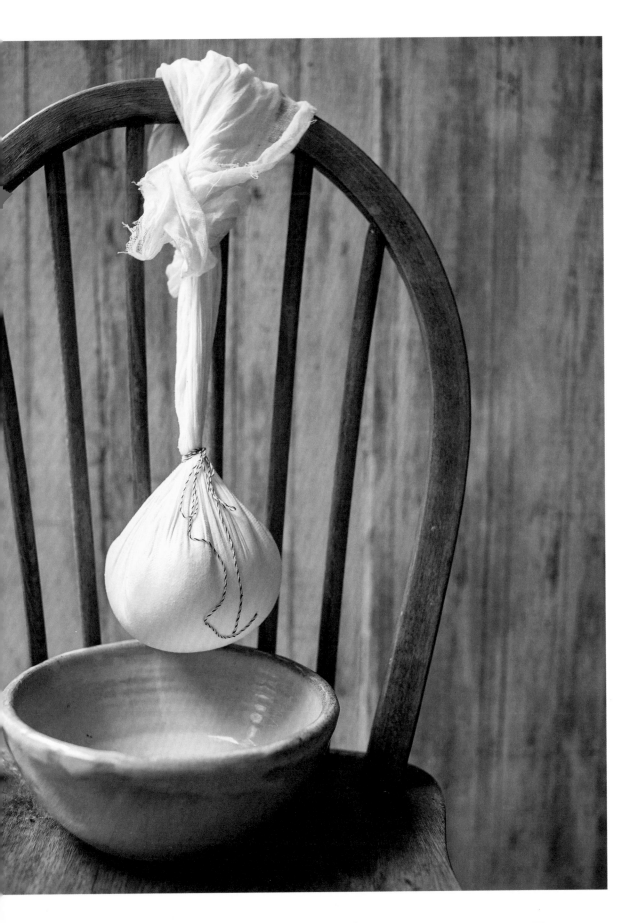

HOMEMADE BUTTER

Making butter is much easier than most people realise, and, as with yoghurt, is rewarding and impressive. My mum would regularly buy gold-top milk from the milkman and pour the cream top into a frappé shaker for us to shake into butter. We loved it, such a treat! As a kid I thought our frappé shaker was magical; now I just think our mum was and still is the coolest.

MAKES AROUND 450G
—

12 ice cubes

1 litre double cream *(the best quality you can buy)*

sea salt

Fill a large jug with cold water and the ice cubes. Leave it to one side. Pour the double cream into the bowl of a free-standing mixer, making sure the bowl is squeaky clean. (You could use a mixing bowl and an electric hand whisk, just be prepared to stand and hold it for a while.) Start by whisking on a low speed, gradually increasing to high. Whisk for around 6–7 minutes, until the cream has clearly split into butter solids and buttermilk. Using clean hands or a sieve, scoop the butter solids out of the bowl and squeeze out the buttermilk (keep this, though, as it will make delicious breads, cakes and dressings – check out the caraway and honey buns on page 232 or my garden salad on page 170).

Place the butter solids in a large bowl and pour over some of the ice-cold water. You want to rinse the buttermilk off the butter solids and squeeze the solids together to form a ball. Pour away the water and repeat a few more times, rinsing and squishing until the water is completely clear. Season with salt to taste, and there you have it, homemade butter! I like to roll mine into a log and wrap it in greaseproof paper. Or you could store it in a ceramic dish – whatever you like.

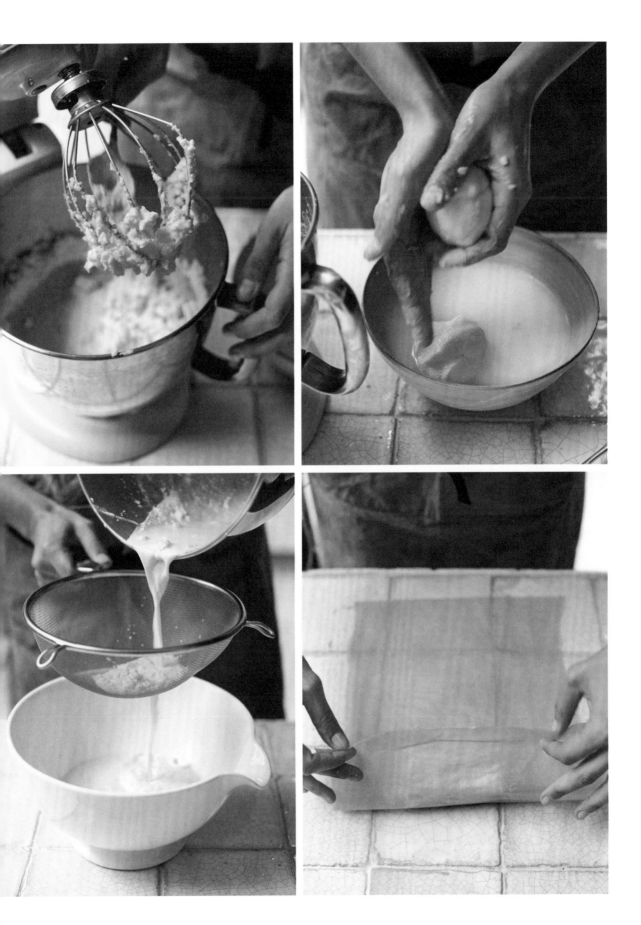

PUMPKIN SEED BUTTER

A hugely popular alternative spread for your morning toast (or rippled into yoghurt, or as the base of a dip), nut and seed butters are so easy to make, and it is much cheaper than buying them already made. I absolutely love proper butter and this is by no means an alternative – how can you compete! But it is delicious in its own right. Also it's a great way of getting some good oils into your diet.

MAKES AROUND 400G
—

300g pumpkin seeds

50g extra virgin olive oil

3 tablespoons maple syrup

a couple of pinches of sea salt

Preheat the oven to 180°C/gas 4.

Scatter the pumpkin seeds on a baking sheet and roast in the oven for 8–10 minutes, until lightly golden and toasted. Remove from the oven and leave to cool, then pour into a food processor. Blitz in the processor for 5 minutes, until you have a smooth paste. You'll need to stop a few times and scrape the mixture down the sides with a spatula. When it is completely smooth, add the remaining ingredients and blitz again to combine.

Decant into a jar and pop into the fridge. Try using it on toast, as a dip, in cakes …

PROPER CUSTARD

Custard doesn't need much of an introduction; whether it's Bird's or made just using egg yolks and cream, everyone seems to have their favourite. This is mine. Laced with vanilla, thick and creamy but not too rich. There really isn't much in life that is better than a helping of Praline Orchard Pie with Bourbon on page 204 with a jug of proper custard.

MAKES JUST OVER 600ML
—

300ml full-fat or semi-skimmed milk

300ml single cream

1 vanilla pod

5 large egg yolks

1 tablespoon cornflour

2 heaped tablespoons golden caster sugar

Pour the milk and cream into a heavy-based saucepan. Split the vanilla pod lengthways, scrape the seeds into the pan and pop in the pod too. Place on a low heat and very gently bring to a simmer. Don't allow the mixture to boil.

While the milk is on the hob, whisk together the egg yolks, cornflour and sugar in a large mixing bowl. When the milk is ready, remove the vanilla pod from the pan and gently pour the hot milk into the bowl with the whisked egg yolks, whisking continuously so they don't scramble.

As soon as it is all incorporated, pour the custard back into a clean pan on a low heat. Stir constantly, and let the custard gently thicken. When it coats the back of your wooden spoon, it's ready. Pour into a jug and serve straight away. If you aren't serving the custard straight away be sure to cover the top of the custard with a piece of cling film, to stop a skin forming. When you want to reheat it, pour it in to a heatproof bowl, and warm over a pan of simmering water.

HIGHLY ADDICTIVE SEA SALT CARAMEL

Does what it says on the tin – the most versatile (and addictive) of baking ingredients.
Homemade sea salt caramel can transform many a cake and pudding.

MAKES JUST UNDER 500G
—

100g unsalted butter

225g caster sugar

130ml double cream

1 teaspoon sea salt *(Maldon or Halen Môn are great)*

Cut the butter into cubes. Pour the sugar into a wide heavy-based pan and place on a medium heat. Melt the sugar without stirring (otherwise it will crystallise), and give the pan a swirl to melt it gently and evenly. Once all the sugar has melted and is a deep golden colour, dot in the cubed butter. It will bubble up, so swirl the pan gently but quickly until all mixed together. Pour in the double cream and whisk it into the caramel until it is all incorporated. Remove from the heat and stir in the salt.

Pour into a bowl, jar or sealed container and leave to cool completely. Cover and store in the fridge for up to 2 weeks.

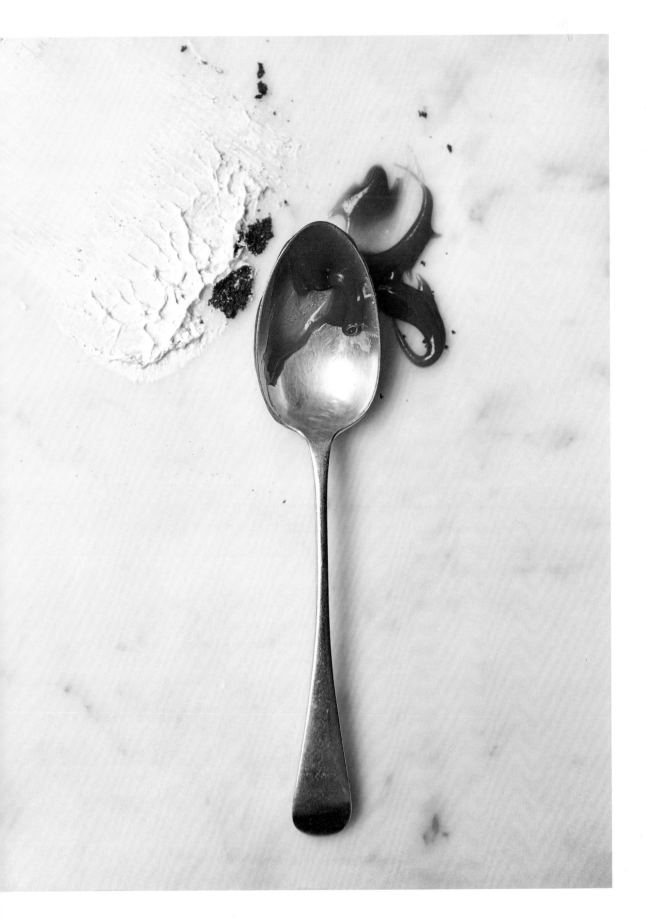

CLASSIC STOCKS

Found in almost every store cupboard, stock cubes are a great way of adding flavour to stews, soups, gravies, and so on, but there is nothing quite like making your own. It's not an exact science, and is something quite instinctive. So instead of giving you exact quantities, I want to talk about flavours and methods.

BASE
—

Whether you are making vegetable, fish, poultry or meat stock, you'll need aromatics. I always use a couple of **peeled onions**, **carrots** and sticks of **celery**, all roughly chopped. You'll need about 8 **peppercorns** and a **bouquet garni** – a few sprigs of herbs tied together. Try thyme, bay and parsley stalks for a standard stock. If you want an Asian inspired broth, try herbs and spices such as **coriander stalks**, **lemongrass** and **star anise** in your base – depending on what you are using it for. A thick slice of **ginger** would be great too.

VEGETABLE STOCK
—

Vegetable stock is the only stock where I soften the base first before adding water. Mainly to encourage the caramelised flavours from the onions, and for a slightly deeper flavour. Pour a drizzle of **olive oil** into a large saucepan, pop on to a medium-low heat and sauté your chopped **onions**, **carrots** and **celery** for 10 minutes, until slightly softened but not coloured. At this point I like to add extra veggies. A sliced **leek** adds great flavour, and a large handful of wiped and torn **mushrooms** and a chopped bulb of **fennel** are great additions. Add to the pan with the **herbs** and **peppercorns** (or whatever spices you are adding), fry for a couple of minutes, then pour in 1 litre of water. Bring to the boil, cover with a lid, then reduce the heat to low and leave to cook for 1 hour. Remove the pan from the heat and leave to cool completely before straining.

FISH STOCK
—

Fish stock is incredibly simple to make. Simply place 600g of **fish bones**, **offcuts** and/or **shellfish shells** in a large saucepan. Add the base ingredients (for fish stock I like to replace one of the onions with a **fennel bulb**) and cover with lots of cold water. Bring to the boil, skim off any scum that comes to the surface, then reduce the heat to low and simmer very gently for 30 minutes – you don't want to cook it for too long, otherwise it will become bitter. Strain through a fine mesh sieve and either leave to cool and pop the stock straight into the fridge, or, for a more concentrated stock, place it back on the hob over a medium heat and reduce it down further. Once refrigerated, use within 3 days, or freeze.

MEAT STOCK

—

For a meat stock you want a rich, deeper flavour, so I'd always roast raw bones first. Mix 1.3–1.5kg of **meat bones** and **offcuts** with the roughly chopped **onions**, **carrots** and **celery** in a roasting tray and pop into the oven for 40–45 minutes, at 200°C/gas 6, until browned and gnarly. Transfer everything to a saucepan with the rest of the base ingredients and cover with cold water. Bring to the boil, skimming off any scum that comes to the surface. Reduce the heat to low and simmer very gently for around 5–8 hours, topping up with water if it reduces away too much, making sure the bones are always covered. When your stock is ready, strain through a fine mesh sieve and either cool the stock and refrigerate, or, to give you a more concentrated stock, pop it back on a medium heat and reduce it down further. Cool, then put into the fridge for up to 5 days. Alternatively freeze once cooled.

POULTRY STOCK

—

For a pale, delicate stock, place around 1.3–1.5kg of **chicken or turkey bones** and offcuts into a large saucepan with the **base ingredients** (you could also use the **carcass** left over from a Sunday roast). Cover with water and bring to the boil. Skim away any scum that comes to the surface, then reduce the heat to as low as possible, so that the stock is just very gently ticking away. Simmer for around 2 hours, topping up with water if it reduces too much. Strain through a fine mesh sieve and cool down, or, for a more concentrated stock, reduce down further over a medium heat. Cool and keep in the fridge for up to 5 days. Alternatively, pop into the freezer. For a richer, more intense stock, roast the bones for 35–40 minutes first, as in the meat stock recipe, and continue as above.

PEACH AND BASIL CORDIAL

This cordial is summer in a glass. Perfect for a party, or just to have stored in the fridge for a summer's day; be sure to serve it with lots of ice and sparkling water.

MAKES 1 LITRE
—

6 peaches

7 lemons

250g caster sugar

12 basil sprigs, plus extra leaves for garnish

sparkling water, to serve

Halve the peaches, remove the stones, and chop the flesh into 2cm pieces. Place in a large pan and finely grate in the zest of 3 of the lemons. Stir in the sugar and basil sprigs, then top with 500ml of water. Place the pan over a medium heat and simmer for 5–10 minutes, stirring until the sugar has dissolved. Leave it to simmer, but don't let it boil, until the fruit is completely soft. Mash the fruit with a potato masher to help it cook right down, and leave it simmering for a further 5 minutes, or until the mixture has thickened a little. Then remove it from the heat and set it aside to cool.

Once the fruit mixture has cooled completely, strain it through a coarse sieve into a mixing bowl, discarding all the solids. Squeeze in the juice from the lemons and stir to combine.

Pour the cordial into a large jug or sterilized bottle. Store in the fridge, undiluted, for up to a week. To serve, pour around 50ml of cordial into a glass (tweak depending on how strong you like your drinks/how tall your glass is) and top up with sparkling water.

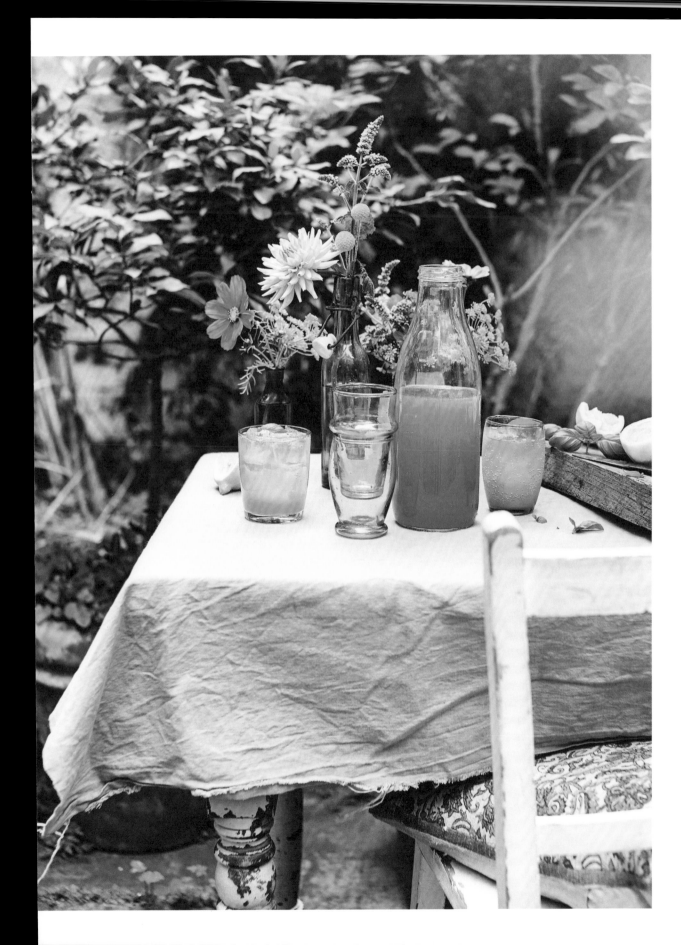

MY SPECIAL MINT TEA
TURMERIC, LEMON AND BLACK PEPPER TEA

My special mint tea infusion is calming, warming, and perfect after a heavy meal. Everyone I make this for is a convert, even my mint-tea-hating sister. Fresh turmeric might sound like a difficult thing to get, but you'd be surprised – seek out a good Indian supermarket and you'll find this peculiar-looking little root in the veg section. It looks like a smaller, orangey-brown piece of ginger. Treat it the same way, peeling it by scraping with a teaspoon to reveal the vibrant root underneath. (Be warned though – it stains!) Try to use it whenever you can, as turmeric is incredibly high in iron, which we need to make red blood cells. These quantities are easily multiplied and if you are making them for more than one, they are even nicer made in a teapot.

MINT TEA, SERVES 1

—

2 sprigs of mint

1 heaped teaspoon good-quality honey

1 teaspoon orange blossom water

Wash and trim the mint sprigs and place them in your mug. Fill the mug with just-boiled water and leave the tea to steep for a minute before stirring in the honey and orange blossom water. Such a delicious after-dinner drink.

TURMERIC, LEMON AND BLACK PEPPER TEA, SERVES 1

—

a 2cm piece of turmeric

½ a lemon

1 heaped teaspoon good-quality honey

a good pinch of ground black pepper

Peel and finely grate the turmeric into your mug, squeeze in the lemon juice and add the rest of the ingredients. Fill the mug with just-boiled water and give it a good stir to dissolve the honey. By the time it's at drinking temperature your tea should be bright yellow and packed with goodness.

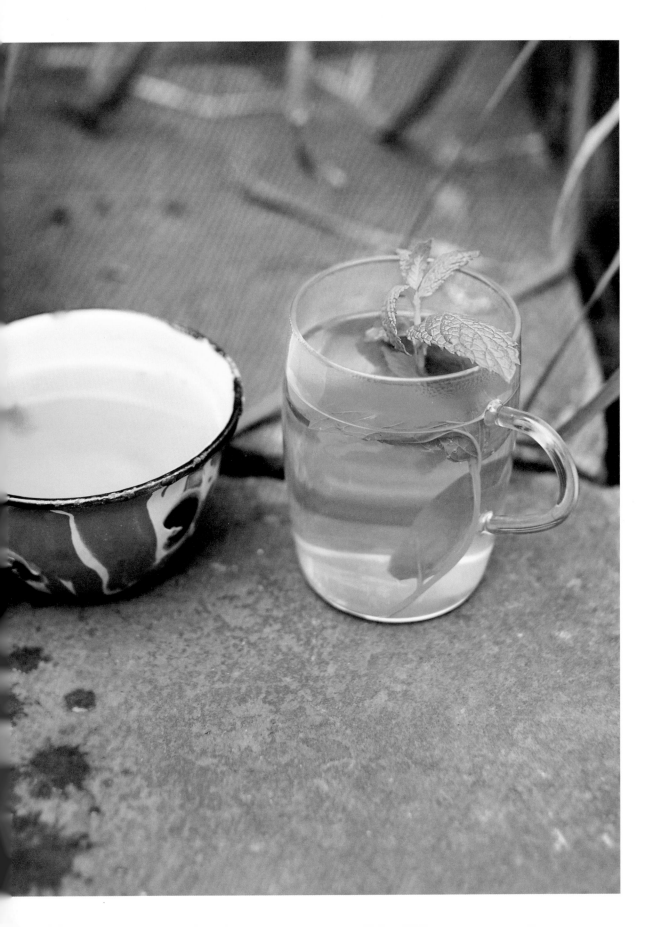

ENGLISH COUNTRY GARDEN PUNCH

Everyone loves a cocktail party, but if you're the host you want to be concentrating on the guests and not constantly making drinks. This garden punch is a winning solution, it's delicious, delicate and refreshing and works wonderfully when made in a batch.

SERVES 14

—

600ml soda water

1.5 litres good-quality apple juice

edible flowers *(optional)*, such as
   rose petals, violets and pansies

250ml elderflower cordial

400ml gin

100ml limoncello *(triple sec also
   works really well)*

3 lemons

½ a cucumber

½ a bunch of mint

The day before you want to serve your punch, put the soda water and apple juice into the fridge to chill, and if you want to make things extra special, prepare some flower ice cubes. Line two ice cube trays with the flowers (alternatively you could use mint leaves, or fruits such as grapes, gooseberries or strawberries). Use boiled and cooled water to fill the trays and pop them into the freezer – this will give you clear ice cubes for maximum effect.

When you are ready to serve your punch, mix the cordial, gin, limoncello and apple juice in a large punch bowl. Finely slice the lemons, and slice the cucumber into ribbons with a potato peeler. Pick the mint leaves and add everything to the bowl along with the soda water. Pop in the flower ice cubes (or ordinary ice cubes) and you're ready to go.

Alternatively, mix the punch and serve it in large jugs with the garnishes in bowls on the side. Let everyone fill their glasses with ice, cucumber, mint and lemon and top up with the pre-mixed punch.

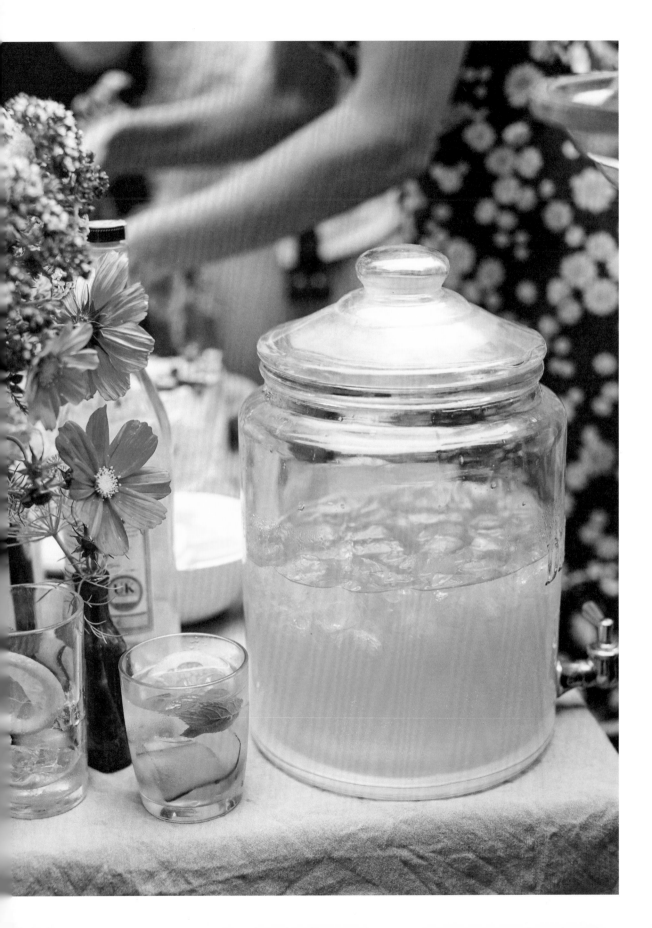

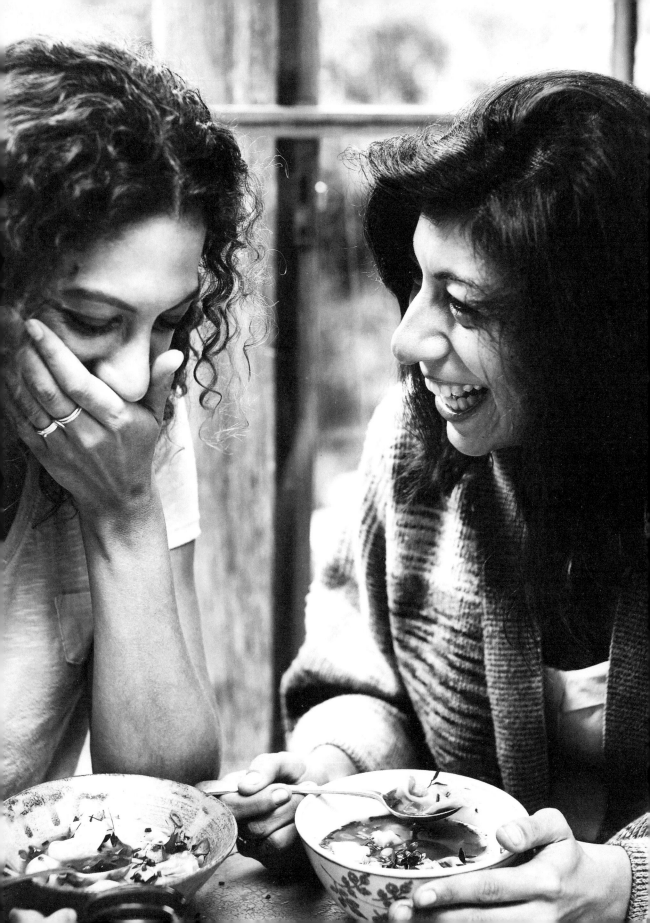

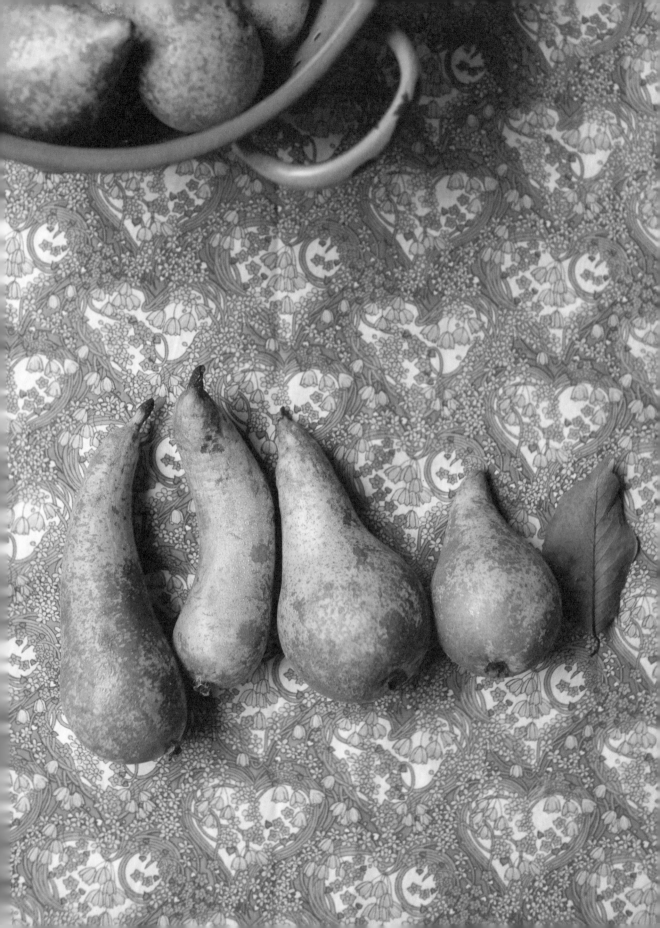

DUKKAH

You'll find dukkah in the spice aisle of most supermarkets now. However, if you struggle to get hold of it, or just fancy making your own, it's dead easy to make. It lasts ages and is fantastic sprinkled on almost anything, especially eggs. Also, let's be honest, homemade really is best.

MAKES AROUND 250G

—

100g blanched almonds or
    hazelnuts *(or a mix)*

100g sesame seeds

2 tablespoons cumin seeds

2 tablespoons coriander seeds

1 teaspoon fennel seeds

1 heaped teaspoon sea salt

1 tablespoon freshly ground black
    pepper

Preheat your oven to 180°C/gas 4.

Spread the nuts in a tray and roast in the oven for around 4 minutes, until lightly golden. Pour them into a bowl and leave to one side to cool.

Toast the sesame seeds in a dry frying pan until golden, then spoon into a bowl and leave to cool. Toast the cumin, coriander and fennel seeds for a minute or so, until they start to smell wonderful, then remove them from the heat.

Once all the nuts and seeds have cooled, either grind them using a mortar and pestle, or pulse them in a food processor with the salt and pepper until you have a coarse blend. Et voilà! Homemade dukkah.

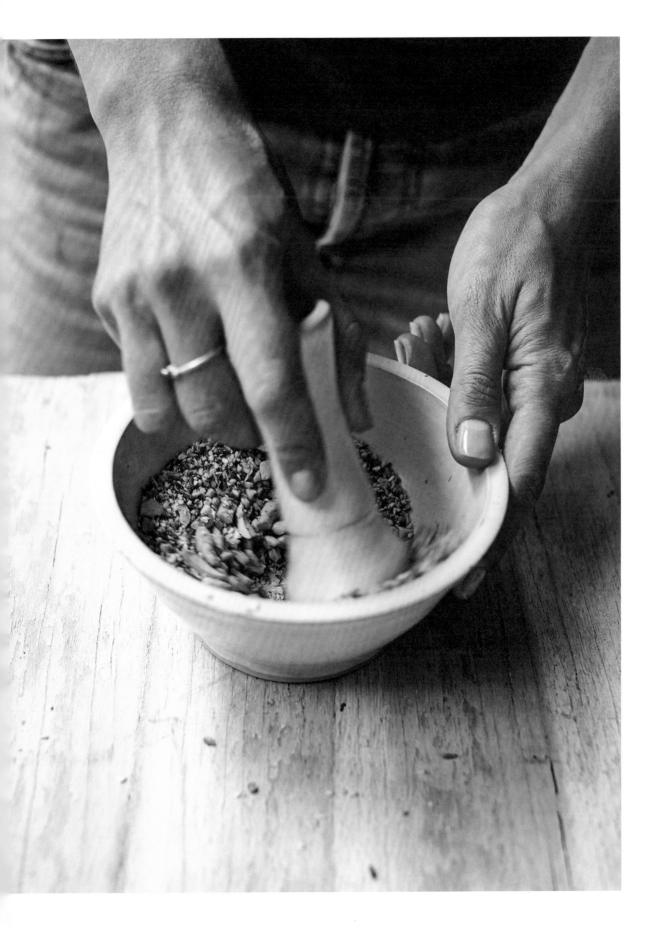

HOMEMADE MUSTARD

So incredibly easy, homemade mustard is an absolute must – it transforms any kitchen. It keeps for ages and makes a great gift, and it goes with everything.

MAKES AROUND 350G
—

100g mustard seeds (*I use a mixture of colours, but if you can only get yellow that'll work too*)

2 teaspoons sea salt

125ml white wine or good cider

100ml white wine or cider vinegar (*match the vinegar to the alcohol you use*)

1 heaped tablespoon runny honey

2 sprigs of tarragon

Place the mustard seeds, sea salt, alcohol and vinegar in a mixing bowl and stir well. Cover, then leave to sit for 48 hours in a dark spot. The seeds will swell up, so make sure you give them enough space.

When you're ready to make the mustard, put the mixture into a food processor with the honey. Pick the tarragon leaves and add these to the mixture, then blitz until you have a smooth paste. Sterilise the jar you are going to store the mustard in (see page 238 for instructions), then spoon it in and seal. Pop the jar into the fridge and leave it for at least 2 days before using. Mustard keeps really well, and will sit happily in the fridge for a couple of months at least.

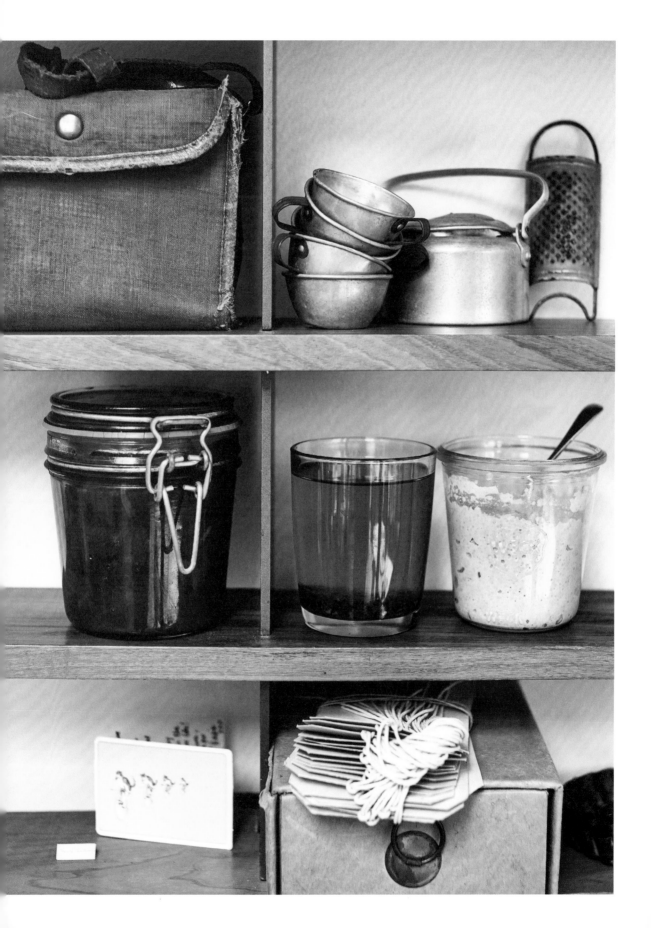

THE PERFECT CHEESE SARNIE CHUTNEY

I adore chutneys and pickles, so much so that they often don't last very long in our house and get eaten straight out of the jar (my husband finds this gross – I think it's a better snack than a bar of chocolate). And this is a great base chutney recipe which can be tweaked depending on what is in season.

MAKES AROUND 1KG

—

100g dates

250g plums

4 garlic cloves

4 red onions

1kg apples and pears

3 tablespoons tamarind paste

a stick of cinnamon

6 cloves

1 fresh bay leaf

1 teaspoon ground white pepper

1 tablespoon sea salt

200g soft light brown sugar

150g granulated sugar

500ml cider vinegar

Remove the stones from the dates and plums. Chop the dates finely and cut the plums into 1cm pieces. Peel and finely slice the garlic and onions. Halve the apples and pears, remove the cores and chop a little larger than the plums.

Place all the ingredients in a large heavy-based saucepan and pop on to a medium heat. Gently bring to the boil, stirring often. As soon as the mixture begins to bubble, reduce the heat to low and leave to tick away, uncovered, for around 2 hours, stirring occasionally so it doesn't stick to the bottom of the pan. The chutney is ready when you drag a spoon through it and the groove doesn't fill with liquid. It should be evenly thick and jammy in texture.

Carefully spoon into sterilised jars (see page 238 for instructions) and seal. You can eat it straight away if you like, but it tastes even better if left for a month or two in a cool dark cupboard.

ADDICTIVE ROASTED CHILLI OIL

Having a cracking chilli oil recipe up your sleeve is a must. It can transform the most simple of meals, acting as a dressing for steamed veg, for finishing pizzas, for drizzling over soups ... This is my pimped-up version with a wonderful heat and slight nuttiness. I urge you to give it a go.

MAKES 500ML
—

2 fresh red chillies

4 garlic cloves

1 tablespoon dried red chilli flakes

1 teaspoon Szechuan peppercorns

1 teaspoon sea salt

1 teaspoon ground black pepper

1 tablespoon sesame seeds *(a mixture of white and black would be ideal, but if you can't get black just use white)*

500ml flavourless oil *(rapeseed or groundnut are best)*

Remove the stalks from the chillies and roughly chop. Peel the garlic cloves. Place them both in a food processor along with the dried chilli flakes, Szechuan peppercorns, salt and black pepper and blitz till finely chopped. Spoon into a saucepan with the sesame seeds and pour in the oil. Place on a low heat and gently sauté for 10 minutes, until everything is lightly toasted and golden.

Leave to cool completely, then pour into a clean bottle and seal. It'll last for months.

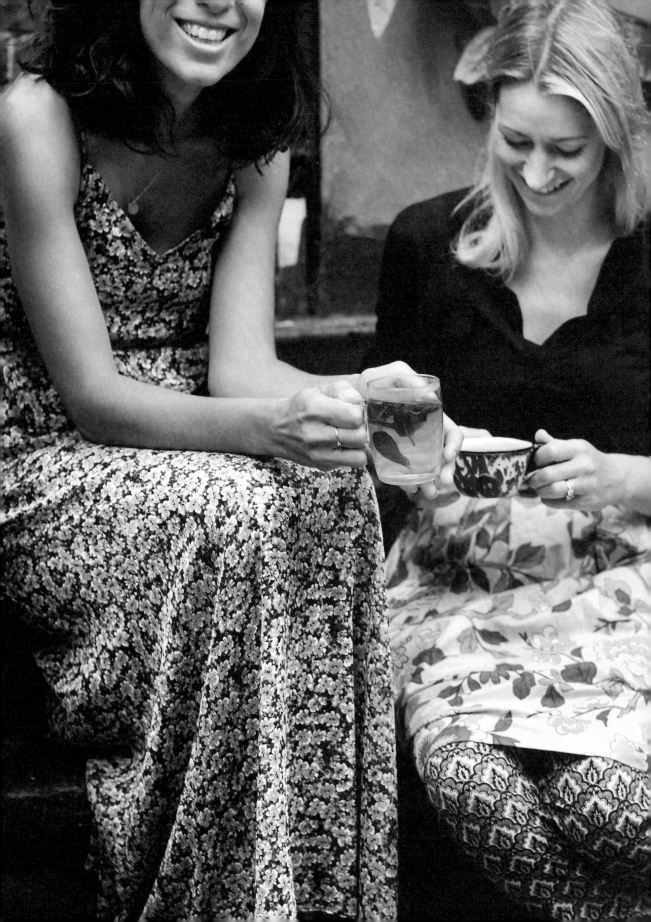

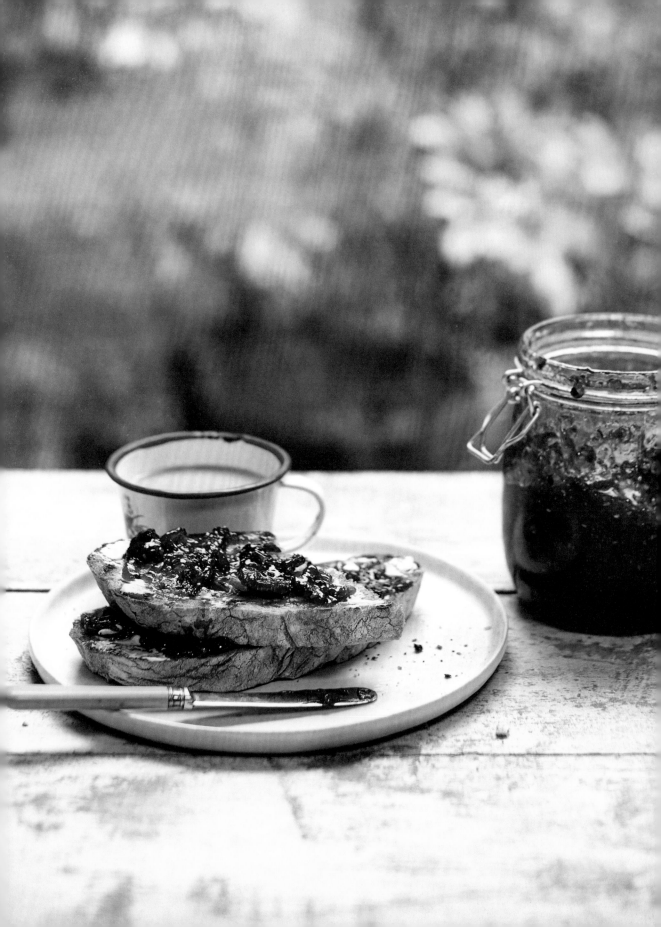

ROASTED MIXED BERRY JAM

I'm a total convert to making my jam this way – it's not the same as the traditional stovetop kind, but for me it's simple and unfussy, and roasting the berries gives them an added depth of flavour that I absolutely adore.

MAKES JUST UNDER 1KG
—

1kg mixed berries

650g golden granulated sugar

1 vanilla pod

1 lemon

Preheat your oven to 180°C/gas 4.

Hull any strawberries and cut any larger berries in half, so that they are all of a similar size. Place in a roasting tray and sprinkle over the sugar. Halve the vanilla pod lengthways, and scrape the seeds into the tray. Halve the lemon and squeeze in the juice and toss everything together well. Nuzzle in the vanilla pod and pop the tray into the oven.

Remove after 30 minutes and carefully mash everything with a potato masher, give it a good stir, then return to the oven. Roast for a further 30–40 minutes, until the berries and sugar have cooked down, and any tops poking out look a little gnarly. (The time will depend on how juicy your fruit is, so check it every 10 minutes.) Remove the tray from the oven, mash the fruit a little more, then carefully ladle into sterilised jars (see page 238). Seal, and leave to cool. Unopened, the jam will keep for months. Once you have opened it, store in the fridge.

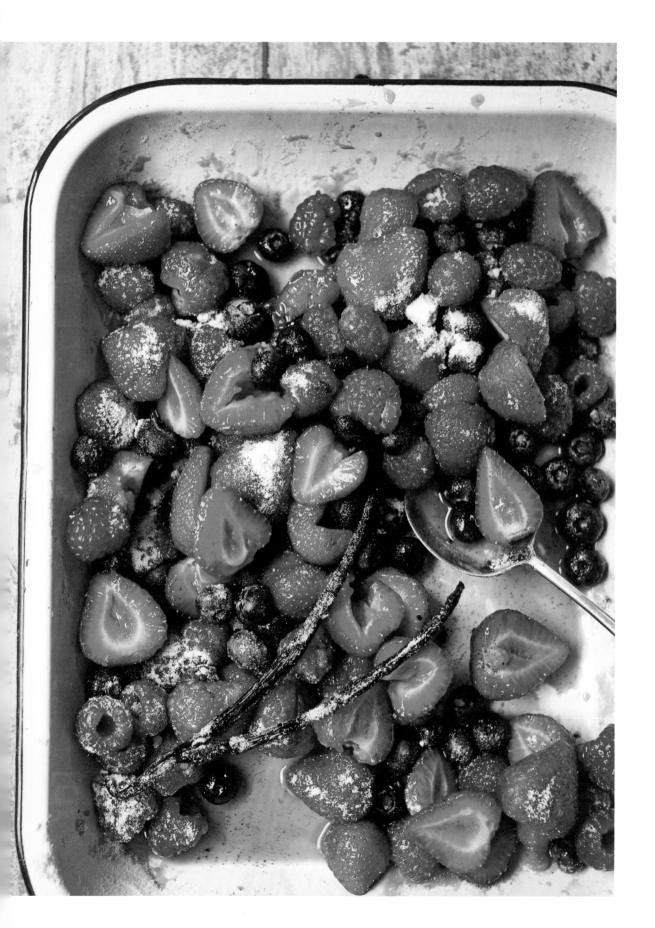

Cheesy as it sounds, writing this book has been a dream come true. It's been empowering, invigorating and emotional all at the same time.

The idea that someone, somewhere, might follow one of my recipes and enjoy my food blows me away, so thank you to every single one of you for purchasing this book and to everyone who has supported me along the way. It means a lot. I hope you love it as much as I do.

To Pete, I think you are incredible and I am so thankful to have you by my side. Thank you for listening to my constant chatter, my wild ideas – good and bad! – for trying my recipes, even when you're so full you could burst, and for being the best friend a girl could ask for. You are my rock, and I couldn't have done any of this without you and your support. I love you.

Rowan, thank you for taking a chance on me, for getting it and understanding what I wanted to say – I appreciate it no end. And for all your knowledge and hard work; I love what we have produced and feel very lucky to have had such creative freedom. It's been inspiring from start to end.

Laura Edwards, the girl with the vision – who'd have thought all those years ago, when we were both eager assistants, that we'd be making books together! Thank you for being so dedicated and for pouring your talent into *Stirring Slowly*. Your pictures leave me speechless – and we know that doesn't happen often. I think you are the bee's knees. Isla, now the shoots are over I feel like I've lost a limb! Thank you for being such a brilliant assistant/right-hand woman and for being a truly wonderful friend. I'm going to miss our Toffee time. To the rest of the shoot crew – Kendal, Vinny, Sam, Abi, and Anna – thank you all so much for your hard work and for being so enthusiastic and kind. Our shoot days have been some of my favourite days, so thank you all for helping make them so much fun. Also, Anna, you have gone down as being the most efficient prop carer I've ever met!

Adrienne, I feel so privileged that you agreed to work on this book and I appreciate every thought and idea you have had – your talent is truly astounding. I can't believe how many happy tears there have been over font choices and page proofs! Thank you for executing it all so beautifully.

Annie Lee, I knew I was in safe hands with you on board! Thank you for being so enthusiastic. To Susannah Otter and Marion Moisy, thank you for going through it all with the finest-tooth comb, for being so enthusiastic (and testing recipes in your spare time!). It's been wonderful to work with you all.

Elly James and Heather Holden-Brown, the kindest agents a girl could ask for. Thank you for standing by me and for helping me find my way. To Claire Postans for the push and encouragement all those years ago, and for being such a wonderful friend. I value your friendship enormously.

My amazing work family – Jamie Oliver, thank you for all your support over the years and for being such a stellar boss and mentor. It's a real honour to work with you, and I have you to thank for so much. Ginny Rolfe, thank you for seeing potential in me all those years ago and for teaching me all you know – you are the style queen! To nutrition goddess Laura Matthews, thank you for taking the time to go through the book with me – and for teaching me about the perils of coconut oil! Abi Fawcett, Sarah Tildesley, Christina Mackenzie, Phillippa Spence, Jodene Jordan, Maddie Rix, Elspeth Meston, Rachel Young, Jo Lord, Rebecca Verity, Pete Begg, Bobby Sebire, Helen Martin, Laura James, Athina Andrelos and Else Grant, thank you for being the dreamiest of dream teams and such wonderful friends. To my extended work family too: Jools Oliver, Gennaro Contaldo, David Loftus, Anna Jones, Andy Harris, April Bloomfield. Thank you for all your encouragement and friendship, it's such a privilege to work with you all.

To Sarah and Ewan, thanks for being incredible testers and always game! And to my mum, Rozzie, Holly, Sarah T, Jo, Lulu, Rebecca, Christina – all my wonderful family and friends who tested my recipes in their spare time – your input has been invaluable! I owe you all big time. And Holly, thank you for not only being a fantastic friend and tester, but for also always being up for a bit of food geekery. I love our chats.

Claire Cain, Laura McKendry, Emma Byrne, Hannah Galvin-Horne, Sophia Brown, Nicole Bacchus – thank you for being the best friends a girl could ask for. I don't know what I would do without friends like you in my life; I feel very lucky.

To Jo and Daf, Trish Ashton, Jenny Halse and all the inspiring SANDS parents I have met along the way – having people reach out is priceless, you have all helped keep me afloat and I think you are amazing.

To Daisy Cooper, thank you for letting me borrow so many of your stunning ceramics for my book! (I'm still your biggest fan.) To Gill at Sytch Farm, thank you too, for all your support along the way. Sophie at Grain and Knot, thank you for the gorgeous spoons.

And last but by no means least, my family. Thank you for never thinking my ideas were too crazy, for putting up with me over the years, and for the unconditional love. Mum thank you for always cooking with us. If it wasn't for your love of cakes I don't think I'd love baking as much as I do! Dad, thanks for all the constructive criticism! I'll get a 10/10 one day. Lulu, thank you for being so supportive and always having my back. To Yiayia, Bahpoo, Lala and Cassie - thank you for making up the motley crew that is my family, and for letting me test stuff on you over the years. We are a strong unit. To my extended family: Carl, Heather, Adam, Myles and Clara, thank you for welcoming me with open arms. And finally thank you to Archie. You have taught me more about the world than I ever could have taught you.

ABOUT GEORGINA HAYDEN

—

Georgina is a cook, food writer and
stylist from North London.

Growing up above her grandparents'
Greek Cypriot taverna in Tufnell Park,
she developed a love of cooking from the
recipes passed down to her. At university
she studied Fine Art after which her passion
for food landed her a job as a food writer and
stylist on various food magazines. She went
on to join Jamie Oliver's food team where
she has worked for ten years. She writes,
develops and styles for magazine features,
books, television projects and campaigns.

Georgina's work is inspired by her visual
eye and her love of travel. Be it sourcing
props at flea markets, travelling the world
for street-food, or cycling round London with
her camera in tow, she documents her food
adventures on her blog. *Stirring Slowly* is
her first book.

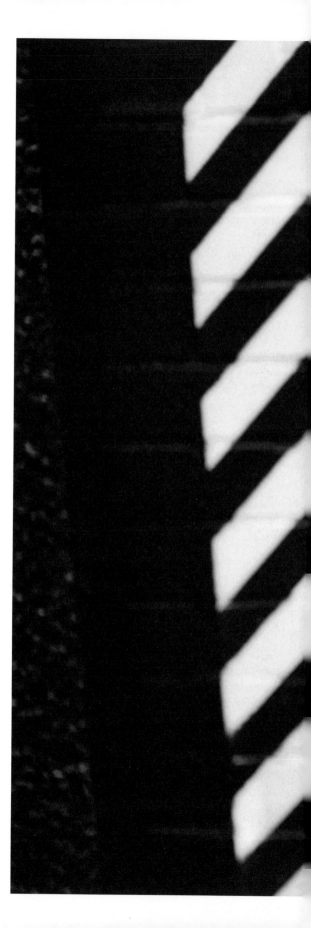

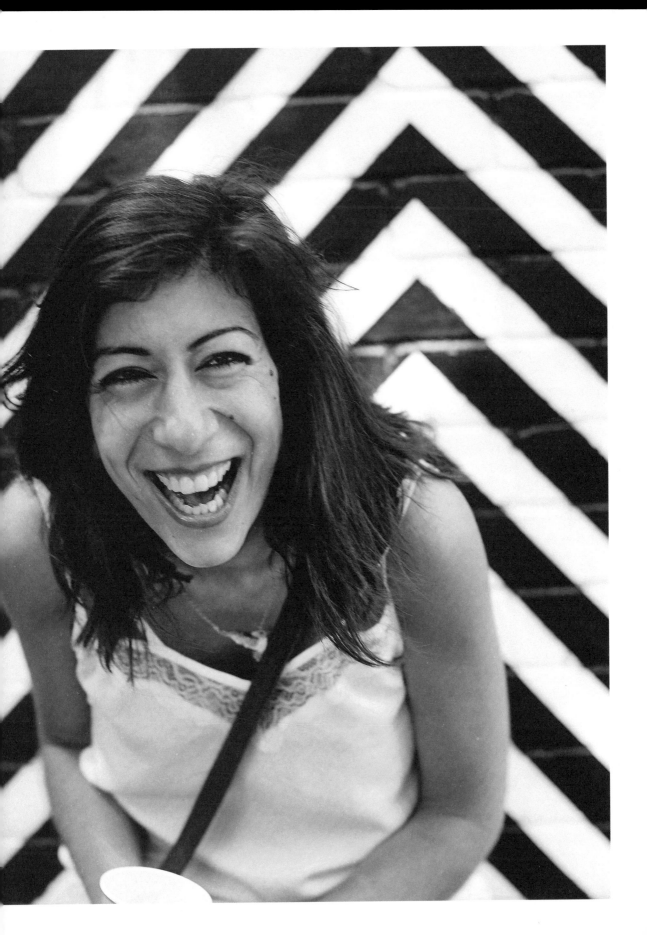

10 9 8 7 6 5 4 3 2 1

Square Peg, an imprint of Vintage,
20 Vauxhall Bridge Road, London SW1V 2SA

Square Peg is part of the Penguin Random House group of companies
whose addresses can be found at global.penguinrandomhouse.com

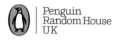
Penguin
Random House
UK

First published by Square Peg in 2016
www.vintage-books.co.uk

A CIP catalogue record for this book is available from the British Library

ISBN 9780224101653
Ebook ISBN 9781473524149

Design by Adrienne Pitts
Photography by Laura Edwards
Props and food styling by Georgina Hayden
Food Assistance by Isla Murray

Printed and bound in China by C&C Offset Printing Co. Ltd.

Penguin Random House is committed to a sustainable future for our
business, our readers and our planet. This book is made from Forest
Stewardship Council® certified paper.

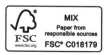